TRANSITION DENIED

of related interest

Written on the Body
Letters from Trans and Non-Binary Survivors of
Sexual Assault and Domestic Violence
Edited by Lexie Bean
Foreword and additional pieces by Dean Spade, Nyala Moon,
Alex Valdes, Sawyer DeVuyst and Ieshai Bailey
ISBN 978 1 78592 797 3
eISBN 978 1 78450 803 6

To My Trans Sisters
Edited by Charlie Craggs
ISBN 978 1 78592 343 2
eISBN 978 1 78450 668 1

The Gender Agenda
A First-Hand Account of How Girls and Boys are Treated Differently
Ros Ball and James Millar
Foreword by Marianne Grabrucker
ISBN 978 1 78592 320 3
eISBN 978 1 78450 633 9

How We Treat the Sick
Neglect and Abuse in Our Health Services
Michael Mandelstam
ISBN 978 1 84905 160 6
eISBN 978 0 85700 355 3

TRANSITION DENIED

Confronting the Crisis
in Trans Healthcare

Jane Fae

Foreword by Amanda De Courcy

Jessica Kingsley *Publishers*
London and Philadelphia

First published in 2018
by Jessica Kingsley Publishers
73 Collier Street
London N1 9BE, UK
and
400 Market Street, Suite 400
Philadelphia, PA 19106, USA

www.jkp.com

Library of Congress Cataloging in Publication Data
A CIP catalog record for this book is available from the Library of Congress

British Library Cataloguing in Publication Data
A CIP catalogue record for this book is available from the British Library

ISBN 978 1 78592 415 6
eISBN 978 1 78450 778 7

Printed and bound in Great Britain

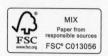

CONTENTS

A Mother's View

Who was Synestra? If you live in North Herts, and if you read the LGBT press, you might have come across her story a couple of years ago. At least, you may have read the bare bones of that story. Synestra was a young trans woman who grew up in and around Stevenage, was educated in Letchworth and, in the last years of her life, went to London to make her fortune, before dying from an accidental drugs overdose at the unspeakably early age of 23.

So much promise, so much heartbreak. At school, she challenged rigid views of gender and sexuality head on, coming out first as gay, then agender. Rather than reject her, as some schools would, they celebrated her difference and in her final year, she was elected head 'boy'. Online, she built a solid following with her personal vlog and a series of expert broadcasts on make-up.

Though that was only the beginning of her journey. By the age of 20 she identified very clearly as transgender and was desperately seeking help from the NHS with her transition. That help was not forthcoming. Instead, as many trans people before her, she got the runaround: she'd not followed the right pathway, ticked the right boxes. Vital letters went missing. Professional assessments were ignored.

So she did what she needed. She started to pay for the treatments and surgeries she so desperately sought through sex work. That, in turn, took her down the road to drugs: first as recreational habit; later, as dangerous addiction. Bad decisions? Yes. But to Syn, there was an inevitable logic to her lifestyle. Besides, it wasn't as though she wasn't enjoying herself. Her story, as so many trans stories, was complicated. To suggest she played no part in her own downfall would be to erase one half of her. She was brilliant. She was lovely. She was also flawed.

None of which excuses the system failures that left her quite unsupported at key moments in her too short life. In 2015, just as her life seemed to be turning a corner, she went to one more party, diced with drugs one last time, and died.

She is missed by many. Her family. Her friends. Her partner. By the trans community, many of whom saw her as likely to play a strong and influential role in future.

For them, as well as for those who would have liked to know her better, this, warts and all, is Syn's story.

Who was Synestra? She was my daughter, my first-born child, and, like all mothers, I cherished her. The utter horror of learning of her death takes my breath away and stops me in my tracks whenever I recollect it. She is never far from my thoughts. To lose one's child is the most unbearable pain one can suffer; it is not the order of things. It will never happen to me, we think. But sometimes it does...

Her name Synestra means 'at one with the stars'. She chose it herself. This beautiful name seems now as if it were some sort of mysterious premonition.

Synestra made a profound impression on so many people. She was quiet, intelligent, and spoke with an eloquence that belied the stunning impact one felt when first setting eyes upon her. She was a dichotomy.

Synestra did live her short life to the full, as she wanted to live it. She learned, and had the power to learn, like no other person I have ever met. Her father, brother and I found ourselves, like many people who knew her, in total awe, and she was way beyond us in terms of knowledge; in just about any subject one cares to mention.

We certainly had our 'ups and downs'. Coping with such an extraordinarily bright child brings its own issues. But Syn lacked wisdom and experience, the worldly-wise things that as we age, we simply 'know'. Being a very bright child gave Syn empowerment over others, and she became almost megalomaniac in her outlook; impossible to influence and certainly impossible to control.

As parents, we could see the devastating effect that drugs were having upon her during 2014, but we were helpless. We quickly realised that Syn of course was an adult in the eyes of the law, and we had no influence in reporting her issues to the doctors, and had no real idea of where to seek help. Had we done so, would she have taken heed? The simple answer is 'no'. Synestra had to find her own path through her difficulties, and this she was finally doing. She was strong, wilful, and once she decided to put this episode behind her, as the clinics and the specialists noted with amazement, she 'recovered' with astonishing speed. Or did she...?

The tragedy was that she was 'almost there'. She had come through the worst of her dark drug addiction and was following a programme to wellness. We all started to relax. And that is where it all fell apart. I will never be able to forgive myself for not being there for her that last weekend, but in my heart I know that the tragedy that unfolded was the accident that had been waiting to happen. No one could foresee the events that unravelled that fateful night, but that accident took away one of the brightest stars – someone who seemed destined for great things. Now we will never know what could have been.

Synestra touched a lot of people, helped a lot of lives, and the world is a lesser place without her in it.

I take this opportunity to mention a charity that I started following her death Synestra's Community Interest Company

(Synestra's CIC). The purpose of the CIC is to help schools, colleges, and universities become more aware of the transgender community. Life is hard for us all at times, but being 'different' and not conforming with society's view of Boys & Girls has a damning impact on those that are unsure, or simply fall in between society's 'norm'. So let's make all toilets just 'toilets' for example, let's allow kids to wear skirts or trousers, short or long hair and remove this need to conform with an idealistic view of pink or blue children. The most difficult 'nut to crack' is the parents themselves. Teachers are getting it, but parents, no, they're not. All parents are proud of their children, but when we talk about non-conformity relating to gender, one can see the bristling effect immediately. Being transgender is not a disease, not something one catches, it's not a fashion, a fad, or any other such nonsense. People are all 'people' no matter what gender, colour or creed. As a society we manage reasonably well with most prejudices, and my aim is try to help eradicate this one.

Amanda De Courcy

Why Syn? Why Now? Why Me?

It is with a sense of responsibility that I set out to write this book. In part, there is that sense of not wishing to 'get it wrong'.

But then, as author, as journalist and yes, as pedant, that is always with me. And in one sense it matters less – legally – if I get some things wrong because my subject is not here to answer back. 'You cannot libel a dead person' is a mantra much liked by historians and obituary writers alike: none of that tiresome checking; no angry letters if you misrepresent views or dates or, well, pretty much anything.

Except, for me, that is part of what makes this work more – not less – difficult. Because they are not here to speak for themselves, I have added responsibility to get them right. Not just the tiresome factual stuff, but the tone and shade as well.

Will those alive today who knew Synestra – Syn as most call her – recognise her in these pages? Will I capture the living person? Or deliver a caricature? Because the temptation when writing of someone no longer here to put their own side of the story is to deliver a eulogy, sans warts, sans flaws, sans anything that might suggest they were anything less than saintly in their day-to-day life.

It is also tempting to shape Syn's life to fit a particular narrative. Because this book is only half about her. The rest is about the challenges that face others following in her footsteps. Young trans people, struggling to cope with a system that disbelieves them. Worse, even when it does believe them, still denies them aid at point of greatest need.

Syn very definitely fell foul of this system. She was disbelieved when she needed help, and denied support. Ultimately, I feel certain, it was her own unique way of resolving these issues that contributed to her untimely death.

Yet, she was privileged too. Syn attended a good school. Unlike many others, it did not tolerate the bullying of pupils for being different. In the end, it celebrated her difference by electing her as Head Boy.

Her parents are well-off, mostly liberal. Unlike some parents, once they came to understand Syn's necessary journey, they never disowned her, never demanded she conform. Instead they sought to support her on her journey.

So many positives!

If there was a flaw, it lay within Syn herself: a preference for sorting things out without fuss, without involving others; a tendency to work her way through the logic of what she needed to do and then go for it.

Sometimes, that is enough. Sometimes, the wall to be climbed is too high.

This is Syn's story. So I have done my best to draw back and to let her friends and family do the talking for her, and through her own writings, Syn herself.

Alongside this is a great deal of detail about what happens in the wider world. For that I am grateful for input from the wider community, including those who have told their stories. Some of these have been painfully personal. Others illustrate in bloody detail how almost every gain won by trans people has been achieved only in the teeth of the fiercest of fierce opposition.

And then there is the ultimate question: Why me? Why Syn? Why now?

In part I'd put it down to coincidence. Serendipity. Some 20 years ago I moved to North Herts, where Syn grew up. First, and briefly, to Stevenage, where she lived for many years. Then to Letchworth, a place I instantly fell in love with and to which I returned in 2014 after an enforced absence of some years, for medical reasons.

I have a daughter, just a year younger than Syn and who – who knows? – could well have been friends with Syn. In talking to Syn's parents, we found overlap: one of her friends, for a time, was also a close friend of Syn's. I was in the process of moving her into a secondary school in Letchworth when my own health emergency struck. Absent that, she might well have ended up in the same school as Syn – but in the year below.

That, though, is all in the realms of 'what if?' But then I also find myself identifying with Syn in various ways: in her school achievements, in her dealing with difference, and ultimately in the thing that set her – and me – apart, in her transness.

And, sadly, I can empathise with, if never truly imagine the depths of loss of Syn's mum, Amanda.

In the end, as I am always careful to stress, there will always be some persona here. The idea of the absolutely independent, neutral journalist is myth, nothing more. The real trick and, for me, the ethical thing to do, is to acknowledge that nothing is without bias, and to make allowances. Not, as some journalists do, lay claim to some theoretical, impossible detached rational stance.

Author's note

The convention, when writing about individuals within the trans community, is to use the name and gender by which they identify. The use of an individual's 'deadname' – the name by which they were formerly known – is not just highly disrespectful: it can also be very hurtful.

It is very clear that, by the time of her death, Syn/Synestra definitely identified as a woman and her preferred form of address was as here: Synestra, or variants thereon.

At the same time, this is biography: a work of historical record. There will therefore be points at which I will reference previous names, previous genders as appropriate. That is especially the case where Syn herself engaged in such topics: but also is difficult to avoid where others knew Syn only by (one of) her previous names. My apologies if that should give offence: it is done to provide narrative clarity and to highlight that Syn underwent a journey, stopping off en route at a sub-station named 'non-binary' or 'agender' before she finally came to understand who she was. And that, too, is part of her story.

It was also very clear, in talking with her mother, Amanda, that use of Synestra's previous name helped her make sense of Syn's life. When writing about trans individuals, it is common to encounter two very different – and opposite – tropes.

The first, that post-transition, one is the same person as before, albeit a little changed in terms of body and outward gender expression; the second, that everything changes, and the post-transition you is in the end a different person altogether from the pre-transition.

Personally, as with all such simplifications, I believe the reality is more complicated. There certainly are differences before and after; but some of what comes after was always there, just well-hidden (sometimes from the subject themselves). Too, there are stages to post-transition, with the immediate post-transition persona some way removed from what went before. The one certainty, perhaps, is that to generalise is to get it wrong.

In the case of Synestra, her mother initially made a conscious decision to put her old life aside. Quite literally, in fact, as Synestra, pre-transition was transferred to a box in the attic labelled Alex. One side-effect of working on this book has been that the boxes have come out, old memories re-engaged and – Amanda's words – 'it really does feel like talking about an entirely different person'.

That is also why, in places, Syn is referenced by her pre-transition name: because this, for Amanda, is the only way to make sense of events. This is especially true of Chapter 1, covering the first ten years of her life.

Mapping the World of Trans

It is not unusual for a work looking at the lives of transgender people and the issues they face to start with a 'Trans 101', a bit like the one set out below.

Trans 101

Trans/transgender is an umbrella term, describing people who experience the need to present themselves as and/or who identify as other than the gender they were assigned at birth.

Gender dysphoria is a medical diagnosis describing the distress of an individual who experiences incongruence between their gender identity and their apparent physical sex. It may also apply where an individual feels unable to present in the gender role that feels appropriate to them but is not the one commonly expected by their society.

Transition is the process of changing gender presentation. This may involve social, medical and surgical change, though not necessarily all three.

Transsexual is a person who wishes to undergo, is undergoing or has undergone transition. While some trans individuals use this term as a means to identify themselves, it should be noted, however, that others consider it offensive, and therefore it should always be used with care.

Transvestite/crossdresser is an individual who wears clothing attributed to a gender different to the one they were assigned at birth, but does not usually experience the requirement to live permanently in that gender role.

Binary trans people are content to describe themselves as either male or female.

Non-binary individuals experience their gender in a range of more biologically and socially diverse ways than binary people. A range of non-binary gender identifications exist.

Gender variance/gender questioning are terms increasingly used to describe variation from expected gender norms. Individuals may experience gender variance/question their gender in a range of ways, from identifying as agender (without gender) to identifying as a gender, binary or non-binary, at odds with that assigned to them at birth.

Cisgender is a term increasingly used to describe those people who are not trans, in much the same way as 'heterosexual' means 'not homosexual'. The term 'cis', in origin, was a preposition meaning the opposite of 'trans'.

Such checklists are to help guide individuals who are (mostly) not trans through the bewildering array of trans groups and terminology that has exploded onto the world stage in recent years. It performs a dual function. It illustrates how trans encompasses a range of different identities; and, in an environment where people are often unwilling to engage in open debate for fear of saying the wrong thing and giving offence, it is a good jumping off point for using language respectfully.

As far as mapping the territory goes, it is useful to begin with the understanding that trans is not one single thing. It is certainly not the cliché 'man becoming a woman', grappling heroically with surgery, before finally, tragically crashing and burning. Tabloids and sensationalist dramas love this. Trans is about gender identity. It is also about the relationship between an individual and their body.

At some fundamental level all trans people feel at odds with the gender/sex assigned to them by society. Different individuals respond in different ways. Where that sense of dissonant identity is overwhelming, they will take steps to change the way that society perceives their gender. Where dysphoria is strong, they will seek medical intervention to change specific features of their body.

These two aspects of transness are by no means absolutely correlated, any more than the desire to improve physical appearance leads inevitably to cosmetic surgery amongst non-trans people. Some individuals, trans and cis alike, happily spend their whole lives being themselves, without surgical or other intervention. For others, life in a less than perfect body is unthinkable. And while there is much debate to be had over the social origins and the desirability of such attitudes, we live in a world in which they are widespread and in which, broadly, we admit it is a good idea to allow people to have agency over their own bodies.

That might dispel some of the puzzlement of non-trans people, brought up on the idea that there is a single 'right way' to be trans and therefore confused by its myriad manifestations. Are cross-dressers not the same as transexuals? Well, sometimes. There are individuals for whom cross-dressing is sexual diversion, and this association between sexuality and trans is one reason why anti-trans sentiment is keen to depict transsexuality as little more than extended kink.

Yet even that simple dichotomy is more honoured in the breach. There are trans people who would transition if they could. Yet for reasons historic and social, the price of such transition is too great. Divorce. Ostracism. Unemployment. These are all, despite a more liberal legal framework for trans people, real consequences.

Therefore every individual, especially those who come to a realisation that they are trans late in life, must balance the costs and benefits of being true to themselves against the disruption this may create.

Some are able to manage being trans by living it part-time. Many, though, need to live as trans in order to discover what works best for them. It might make sense for some to start out as non-binary or gender questioning, because they cannot make head or tail of the gender assigned them, and over time, a subset of these will realise that transition is the right option for them. Others make the journey in the opposite direction, believing, initially, that a binary transition is the right solution and only later understanding that this creates as many issues as it solves.

It is important to hold on to an understanding of this fluidity when looking at Synestra's life. What is clear is that, from an early age – certainly 12 or 13, but likely earlier – she was grappling with questions of gender identity. For a while, as some trans individuals do, she explained her feelings by viewing herself as gay. That did not last long, and as she matured, she experimented with various models of self. Synestra journeyed from agender, to a-masculine, taking significant steps to suppress male characteristics in her body, to binary trans woman at the time of her death.

Trans ecosphere

If that is the trans eye view of trans, it is equally important to acknowledge that trans does not exist in a vacuum. It exists within the world, within society, within an environment – a political and social ecosphere – that is at best sceptical, at worst outright hostile to the existence of trans people. So in addition to the usual Trans 101, let us take a brief look at that ecosphere and map some of the most significant existential threats to trans people.

For much of their public existence, the trans community has

found itself at the intersection of a particularly vicious pincer movement of interests and ideologies that in most circumstances would be at loggerheads with one another. Unluckily, in trans, they have found a reason for burying their differences and putting the boot in collaboratively.

The story begins with the medical and especially the psychological and psychiatric establishments. As medical and surgical transition became ever more a thing in the 1960s, it became necessary to provide medical justification for clinical intervention. This gave rise to two phenomena. The first was a series of ever more convoluted attempts to explain transness, to give it some sort of theoretical base. Since these early theoretical fumblings came from within the medico-psychological community, it is hardly surprising that they should seek to locate trans within some sort of clinical model of disorder, with clearly defined causes, symptoms, diagnostic criteria and treatments.

Let's pause right there. Because the 'medical model' is widely recognised as problematic when it comes to psychological issues – and not just by psychiatrists such as R.D. Laing, who raised this issue as long ago as 1971. In fact there are two problems. The first lies in the slightly abstract but nonetheless critical sphere of what we mean when we talk about 'illness'.

When it comes to physical ailment, illness is generally understood as some sort of disorder or improper functioning of our bodily systems. We are mostly not 'meant to' spend our days with a streaming nose or uncomfortably high temperature – but note the scare quotes and the philosophical Pandora's Box hinted at in that simple phrase – and therefore we feel justified in regarding illness as something to be put right.

This idea of proper function becomes problematic when the medical profession deals with issues of impairment – another loaded word – either physical or mental. If a person *is* a certain way, either in terms of their body or their mind, there is a strong case that the role of medical science should not always be to fix or 'cure'. Because that way lies a world in which everyone is judged by some impossible normative standard. Any lack of success in achieving that standard is then, to some degree, regarded as personal failure.

If illness is not quite as straightforward a concept as we imagine in respect of the body, how much more difficult when it comes to the mind? Psychology, psychiatry and related disciplines are little more than a century old. In that time, all manner of conditions have been diagnosed as 'disordered', only for a subsequent generation to declare a decade or two later that such-and-such condition was not disordered, but in fact some sort of natural variation in the human condition.

Across the 20th century, each decade seemed to bring forth a new GUT (Great Universal Theory) for cognition, perception, learning – only to sit back and watch as the next decade tore it to shreds.

This is especially the case when it comes to sexuality, where one generation's 'disorder' often turns out to be a simple medicalising of social prejudice. One only has to look at the efforts, once attempted by respected medical professionals, to 'cure' homosexuality to understand this. Thankfully, 'reparative therapy' – the collective name for such efforts when directed at gay people – is now unlawful in many states, and frowned upon in many more. Yet it is still an approach that some psychiatrists are happy to contemplate for trans people, especially younger ones.

The second issue is that the medical model applies only sketchily to issues of the mind. In the case of physical ailments, influenza is clearly caused by a virus. That virus may be observed in the laboratory: it is a physical thing. People know, broadly, when they are suffering from flu: they likely have a fever, cough, sore throat, runny nose. Their body may ache. And while some of these symptoms might mimic symptoms brought about by other ailments – sneezing, for instance, might equally indicate cold or hay fever – medical professionals have enough experience of what flu looks like to be able to diagnose it with reasonable accuracy.

It is also the case that flu responds to certain treatments. Usually that means bed rest and plenty of fluids: occasionally specific anti-viral medication. Not every single bout of flu will be experienced identically by those suffering from it. Still, there is sufficient commonality for us to state, with confidence, that flu is a 'thing'. It exists independently of human theorising.

Compare and contrast depression or anxiety, which are two of the more common psychological ailments diagnosed. Certainly, there is a core of symptoms that, in popular awareness, might be recognised as indicative of these states. Although it requires only a cursory reading of the literature in this area to realise first, that what the medical establishment regards as anxiety or depression is by no means the same as what the general public might consider these to be. Second, professionals differ far more over what constitutes either than they do for flu.

There is no agreement as to causes. Pick a school of psychology and you pick an explanation: different experts give different weight to a variety of causes, including stress, medication, upbringing, genetic factors. Nor do they agree on what treatment to prescribe. Or rather, depending on training, different treatments may be preferred. Again, the literature is awash with studies that show patchy response to different treatments, as well as some possible matching of cure to cause. In other words, while society as a whole may rely on these diagnoses, they are fundamentally different to a diagnosis of flu.

This is especially the case when it comes to any diagnosis of 'being transgender'. Over the years, a variety of models have been advanced to explain transness. Note, again, the preference that many academics have for a Trans GUT: that is, a single all-encompassing theory as to what trans is and why people are trans. Yet, as this book records, there is evidence that trans is absolutely NOT one single thing at all.

The *Diagnostic and Statistical Manual* (DSM), published by the American Psychiatric Association (APA), is pretty much the go-to handbook for the definition of any psychological illness or disorder in the US. It is also influential in other diagnostic tools, such as the World Health Organization's International Classification of Diseases (ICD). Between them these are widely used to categorise what is and what is not mental illness. The DSM initially classified being transgender, which it named gender identity disorder, as a disorder, alongside being gay.

There has since been a long slow march back from these positions. The inclusion of homosexuality as a disorder was partially rescinded in 1973. Yet gay people still had to wait until 1987 for the slur on their sexuality to be removed entirely.

As for trans people, in 2013 the DSM-5 reclassified 'identity disorder' as gender dysphoria. The claim that being trans is intrinsically disordered was abandoned. Now it asserts that the primary cause of discomfort for trans people is the stigma attached and the social consequences of coming out as trans.

The position in respect of the ICD remains muddy. According to a series of official statements by the World Health Organization, being transgender is *not* a mental illness. Its removal from the catalogue of mental illnesses is widely forecast for the next edition of the ICD – its 11th – expected to be published in 2018.

Meanwhile, treatment of individuals diagnosed with dysphoria is mostly subject to standards of care set by the World Professional Association for Transgender Health (WPATH), formerly known as the Harry Benjamin International Gender Dysphoria Association. In addition to setting standards of care, WPATH aims to support clinical and academic research aimed at developing evidence-based medicine in respect of trans people.

Thus, when you read that the standard for treatment of trans individuals includes no gender affirmation surgery before the age of 18, or that prior to surgery, candidates should be assessed by a mental health professional, this – and much else besides – has its origins in the WPATH standards.

There is growing unanimity around the treatment of dysphoria, increasingly based on an assessment of actual social outcomes. At the same time, there remain 'experts' whose primary academic obsession is in providing some sort of 'scientific' explanation for transgender people. In this, a motley assortment of psychiatrists and sexologists appear to owe more to the now discredited theorists of the 19th and early 20th centuries who spent much time attempting to theorise homosexuality – or 'sexual inversion' as it was then classified.

In terms of explanatory models, there have been many attempts to define trans as some variant of homosexuality or same-sex attraction. A difficulty with this categorisation is that trans people do not uniformly demonstrate attraction to the gender to which they were originally assigned. Nonetheless, a number of sexologists have constructed a series of theories that transness, or the phenomenon of trans women, is the result of something called autogynephilia (essentially, being turned on by imagining oneself as a woman).

The approach, for all that it is dressed up in the language of scientific experiment is essentially a-scientific. The theory is unfalsifiable (falsifiability is widely considered essential if a theory is to be considered properly scientific). It is also constantly adjusted to maintain its 'truth' when presented with contradictory evidence.

Once located in clinical space, the next step was pretty

much inevitable. Trans became a medical specialism: the only people qualified to understand it properly were clinical experts. They would henceforth act as both gate-keepers to treatment, determining who was worthy of it, as well as arbiters of what treatment should consist of.

The idea that trans people had any expertise in their own condition, or should be allowed a say in how they were treated, was off the agenda for decades. This, in turn, led directly to some egregiously bad treatment of individuals. The clinical establishment imposed rigid ideas of who should be entitled to treatment – principally, individuals likely to transition neatly and unobtrusively within the binary. Trans women were denied access to medical treatment for being too tall, for being married, for refusing to affirm an attraction to men and for a host of reasons besides.

Not that long ago, a trans woman was politely informed by the clinician responsible for reviewing her case that while she was definitely trans, the fact that she had large hands meant she would never 'pass' as female: so he recommended she simply get on with her life and accept nothing could be done. According to this individual, he told her: 'While I have no doubt you are transsexual...I am not going to prescribe hormones for you. Your hands are too big, your feet are too big, your shoulders are too broad and your chin is too masculine; you look like a man in drag. I suggest you get on with your life and try and put this behind you as best you can.'

If admission to treatment was subject to strict rules, so too was continuing treatment. Trans women, especially, were policed as to clothes and posture: women wear skirts and sit 'just so'. And dissent from this view was dangerous: for ultimately, unless you had independent means, not only access to treatment, but your status as a trans person was in the hands of people who were not the least bit trans. Readers may wonder if this reflected a certain inevitable sexism inherent in a situation where mostly middle-aged men got to pontificate on what was sufficiently female behaviour.

Yet let us not forget that this is in essence the same male-dominated medical establishment that, as recently as 1944 was prescribing clitoridectomy, or removal of the clitoris, for women whose sexuality did not conform to their own ideals of propriety.

It is also arguable that as much as 90% of the expert opinion ever pronounced on trans issues has been wrong. One only has to review the differing medical opinions provided in 1960, 1980, 2000 and since to observe that clinical views of what causes an individual to be trans, its manifestation and its treatment have varied so widely over the years that they simply *cannot* all be right. Logically, most of them must have been wrong!

Many reasons, many excuses, were advanced for this gate-keeping. In the early days, and beyond, there was concern that individuals might ascribe to being trans, feelings and desires that in fact arose from some form of mental illness: that they were in fact delusional. That is valid. There are many things that people may opt to do, from writing a will to consenting to surgery, where the start point is they should be of sound mind. In the case of surgery, this extends to a need for informed consent: individuals should be aware of possible adverse consequences of any surgery before signing up for it.

Yet, in respect of trans healthcare, the overriding concern, cited over and over, goes well beyond a basic insistence on informed consent. Medical professionals and pundits alike obsess over individuals making poor/irreversible choices and subsequently experiencing 'regret'. This may be superficially plausible, but it does not survive a millisecond of prodding. Because medical treatments – including those that may be life-saving or come with a high degree of social acceptance – are awash with regret. In the UK, patient surveys suggest that not only treatments for conditions such as prostate cancer, but also abortion, attract higher levels of regret than transition, which, by the same measurement standard, continues to be one of the least regretted procedures carried out in the NHS today.

Even where regret is experienced, further research suggests this may largely be attributed to two factors: the limitations on existing transition procedures (many individuals wish that more could be done); and social factors, including widespread discrimination in many areas against trans people.

So why the concern? A range of factors is likely in play. Gender transition remains well beyond the ken of the majority of the British public. So it is, perhaps, natural that many view it as an extreme and edgy procedure. They cannot conceive the world as seen through the eyes of the average trans person for whom transition – and surgery – are often viewed as minor procedures: little more than the next step on a logical pathway.

Still, with such worries, one might be forgiven for imagining that some medics, fearful of being sued, will play safe. Less forgivable is the way in which regret has been used by a range of individuals who appear to have little interest in the care of trans people, beyond erecting barriers and making life difficult for them. The collective term for this approach is 'concern trolling', broadly defined as the practice of disingenuously expressing concern about an issue in order to undermine or derail genuine discussion.

For concern trolls, no matter whether politically or religiously motivated, regret is a handy stick to beat trans individuals with. So too is the question repeated ad nauseam when dealing with youth transition, of whether individuals are 'too young to know'. Perhaps. However, as discussed in Chapter 1, the consequences of being trans pre-puberty are minimal, so this, too, is a red herring.

Trans predators

What this highlights is that in addition to being policed by medical personnel, trans people have numerous powerful predators out there. These seek to deny trans existence and, where possible, to deny individuals access to appropriate treatment.

This goes beyond those in the medical community who, through an excess of controlling impulse, have often proven fair-weather friends: for some trans people, as much problem as solution. On the whole, though, the medical community has tried, however imperfectly, to support trans people.

One group inimical to trans people from the outset is a disparate coalition centred around tradition, fundamentalist religion and sexual conservatism. As one might expect, this grouping is 'just not having it'. Transgender is against God's order, or, for the non-religious, against the natural order.

That said, an important corrective to this litany of religious inspired hatred is that it does not officially extend to the Catholic Church or even other recognised churches. The Church of England, for instance, voted in 2017 to institute welcoming services for trans people in their new gender identity should they choose to celebrate their 'coming out' in religious form. This may come as a surprise to some who have read, in the LGBT press, how the Pope has supposedly compared trans individuals to the nuclear bomb. But this is a serious misreading of what the Pope has said with regard to official Church doctrine on the matter, which is, according to some highly placed members of that Church, precisely nothing.

There is an ongoing and increasingly heated war being waged with exponents of 'gender theory', which many Christians see as harmful to family values. Academically, gender theory is an offshoot of post-modern and feminist thinking. But nothing has been said about the ethical position of trans people within the Church. The nearest the Pope has come to any pronouncements on this topic is in discussion of individual cases. In one, the Pope spoke of a conversation he had with a trans man: he spoke respectfully using male pronouns, and condemned a parish priest who had disparaged him. In a second instance, the Pope, before his elevation, publicly supported the efforts of a nun who provided aid to a community of trans sex workers.

None of this is to say that in the fullness of time, the Catholic Church will not decide to come out as firmly against trans as it has against gay and bisexual people. Rather, it is to set a limit to the condemnation, and to recognise that religious hatred, insofar as it is sanctioned officially, tends to have its roots in more dogmatic elements of the mainstream. Not just Christian evangelicals, but amongst traditionalists from other religions too: more conservative Jews, more radical Muslims, and so on.

Many of these view being transgender as closely allied to homosexuality, or some variant thereof. Since they view homosexuality as an undesirable perversion, it is not unexpected that their hatred of all things gay transfers out to trans. This, it is often argued, is as good a reason as any for the trans community to remain allied to the wider LGBT community; well, one of two reasons.

The first, positive, is that many LGB individuals, who have suffered much for having a different sexuality, are more likely to understand what it is to be on the receiving end of discrimination for one's gender identity. The second, rather less positive, is that while a trans person may understand the difference between them and a gay individual, the average hater does not. Whether or not haters will direct violence at you is not determined by the finer points of where you sit on the LGBTQI spectrum, but is motivated simply by difference.

If it is to be expected that this group, the reactionary and religious, would be staunchly anti-trans, the second group who have proven in every way as vicious, as assiduous and as hostile as the first is a small but vociferous sub-set of the feminist world. The seeds for this particular brand of anti-trans ideology were sown through the publication of Janice Raymond's *Transsexual Empire* in 1979, which asserted, amongst other claims, that:

- sex is determined by chromosomes: XY is always male; XX always female
- the experience of being raised as a girl and menstruating determines a woman
- transsexualism is caused exclusively by the sex stereotyping of patriarchal society, while those support professionals – surgeons, psychiatrists, counsellors, electrologists, etc. – who persuade 'foolish persons' to change are a secondary reason.

The focus for her onslaught was trans women. She barely considered trans men, otherwise dismissing them as 'the tokens that save face for the transsexual empire'. According to Raymond, the patriarchy introduced sex changes as a means of controlling gender stereotypes, which act in the interests of men. Once extra-natal conception is introduced, she went on, biological women will become redundant. She asserted: 'All transsexuals rape women's bodies by reducing the real female form to an artefact, and appropriating this body for themselves.'

Raymond had little patience for trans women who would support the feminist cause. These 'lesbian-feminists' as Raymond described them, 'show yet another face of patriarchy'. That is, she argued, 'the male-to-constructed-female who claims to be a lesbian-feminist attempts to possess women at a deeper level, this time under the guise of challenging rather than conforming to the role and behavior of stereotyped femininity'. In essence, by assimilating to and within women's protest groups the trans feminist's aim was to supplant true feminists from doing their work.

Raymond's solution was simple. She wrote: 'I contend that the problem of transsexualism would best be served by morally mandating it out of existence.'

The impact of her work in the US was controversial and, according to some, deadly. The National Center for Health Care Technology (NCHCT) co-opted her to write a report on the ethics of trans medical care. Despite subsequent protestations of innocence, it is believed by many in the trans community that Raymond's claim that trans healthcare was ethically controversial would have likely played a major part in having trans medical care routinely excluded from both public and private health insurance plans during the period 1989 to 2013. This, activists have claimed, contributed to the death of hundreds of trans individuals.

In addition to making a significant intervention in the public debate, then still in its infancy, Raymond and a few other mostly self-described 'radical feminists' began a war of attrition against the trans community that continues to this day. Any increase in trans rights is opposed; any improvement in the day-to-day living conditions of trans people is counter-argued. They posit an array of concerns ranging from 'the evidence is not there yet' through to alleged dangers to non-trans women.

The frequent core of this argument is that since men can impersonate trans women, any rights handed to trans women allow predatory men more easily to invade women's spaces. In fact, there is little to no evidence that specific measures granting rights to trans people are massively abused by non-trans individuals. Since approximately 2015, there have been a number of cases in which such intrusion appears to have taken place. Almost all have been instances where some individual – political activist or journalist – has decided to break the law, as these groups claim it can be broken, in order to prove a point.

A little like going out and running over a pedestrian in order to prove that road safety provisions are inadequate.

More recently, Raymond's arguments have received a new lease of life with the claim that trans women can never be women because they did not grow up as such. That claim is ideological, rather than scientific in the strictest sense. If, as some increasingly argue, transness is a variation in the natural self-identification process – learnt in childhood, but mediated by biological process – it is also wrong.

Yet in 2017, the ideological heirs to Raymond's position, despite being a small minority in UK feminist groups, have harried the trans community. They have campaigned against (evidence-based) healthcare for trans children, against recognition of trans people as their identified gender, and they have used their platform in the media to spread harmful myths. Such groups have also worked assiduously to exclude trans women from any groups they deem should be 'women only', including feminist organisations that are otherwise supporting of trans people. On several occasions, they have taken their dispute out onto the street, picketing events they consider too inclusive and publicly accusing trans women of rape.

This war with the rad fems has given rise to a usage that is itself controversial. Many in the trans community use the term 'TERF' – or 'trans-exclusionary radical feminists' – to describe those who work against them, although it seems that this term was invented, in the first place, by feminists seeking to separate their own trans-accepting view from those who were less accepting. This, in turn, has elicited the counter-accusation from those named such that the term is a 'slur' and anti-woman.

The latter seems to be a bit of a stretch: a little like arguing that to call a bunch of right-wing politicians 'racist' is a slur against all politicians, or all men. It is very clear that most of those identified as TERF are radical feminist in their ideology and therefore RF. More debatable is just how trans-exclusionary one needs to be in order to justify the addition of TE.

Raymond, on any criterion, probably qualifies. So, too, do an army of online trolls whose primary function appears to be to pop up and harass trans people whenever the opportunity arises, through dead-naming (using an individual's pre-transition name), mis-gendering (calling trans women men/he, and trans men women/she) and making a range of serious and usually false allegations about them (trans women are described as rapists or rape apologists).

That said, not every individual assigned to the TERF category is radical feminist. In addition, many claim to accept the existence of trans people. When it comes to specifics, though, they are mostly opposed to granting individual rights. In other words, they deny exclusionary tendencies, but the label appears to fit.

I use the term where it feels appropriate. But sparingly. For like any simplification of complex categories, TERF is both handy shorthand and inflammatory declaration. I cannot speak for those who object to being labelled such. There are times, though, when I have observed an individual heap abuse on a trans woman, then squawk outrage at having this four-letter epithet pinned to them. This appears little more than another form of trolling. Outrage trolling, perhaps.

The ultimate irony of the present situation is the ideological convergence between predator groups from right and left. Two groups, viscerally opposed on almost every other issue, have united to attack trans people. In doing so, they appear, at some level, to have fundamentally betrayed the values they stand for. In the first, Christian charity; in the second, protecting women from patriarchal power structures.

There is further irony to be found in the fact that both these groups also attack trans people for being 'activists'. This is clever because, in one sense, it is literally true. Trans people have come from behind, in terms of legal rights and recognition within society. Across the board, in education, employment, and on-street safety, they are disadvantaged if not actively discriminated against.

So trans people campaign. Constantly. Because, they want the same basic rights as everyone else. Campaigning – activism – in this sense is analogous to rights movements of the 60s and 70s. Then, minority groups campaigned for equal rights for those of different race, gender, sexuality. It is not, as it is twisted in some popular representation, some sort of evangelising zeal or recruitment to the 'trans way of life'.

The real aim, for trans campaigners is no different from the goal of most campaign veterans, which is to go home, cultivate one's garden, and to get on with life without the need to fight constantly just to stay still.

Somewhere around the edges of the above is a third problem group. This is ideologically diverse, and, as advocates of free speech and liberal values, appears, on the surface, to contain the sort of people who should be good allies. Many of these are to be found in the media. Their besetting sin, though, is a firm belief in the idea that if only an issue can be debated enough times, then its sting will be drawn and harmony and goodwill will follow naturally.

From this quarter comes a constant pressure for debate of the 'real issues': usually a confected forum in which trans people are put on the spot and required to answer questions that go to the core of their existence.

It may seem outwardly harmless, yet this is to miss the point twice over. In discussing with one of these individuals why constant debate over the existence of a group was justified, they respond by saying that they would not object in the slightest if their own existence was similarly up for debate. Superficially, that is respectable: those who advocate free speech are asking for nothing they do not accept for themselves.

Except. What seems to be missed here is the dimension of privilege. For these individuals, it is never likely to be the case that these debates will impact directly on their lives. A 'debate' about whether we would reduce rates of sexual violence by locking up all male adults from dusk till dawn has edge value. It creates a stir and mainstream media love it. Experienced debaters can enjoy making the case for and against. In the end, though, this is just hot air. It is not going to happen; at least not without a massive shift in cultural values.

Similar debates – for instance, whether trans people should be barred from public loos – are not merely academic. This is happening across parts of the world including parts, such as the United States, previously deemed tolerant, liberal. So this debate matters, in a way that an equivalent debate about another group would not.

Add in two more considerations. The impact on the (mental) health of many trans people of this constant insistence on debate is not negligible. As will be detailed later in the book, many trans people give up going out, give up taking their children out of the house, because of fear that is at least in part generated by the pressure of such constant debate.

That also overlooks the worst effect of this intellectual meandering. It serves, time and again, to empower and, in their minds, justify the actions of bigots, transphobes who then go on to discriminate against trans people or even attack them physically. Often, as a journalist, I pick up reports of an increase in anti-trans violence following milestone/high-profile 'inquiries' by the media.

It is difficult to make the direct connection, but my gut feel, based on years of reporting this stuff is that it is there: it exists.

That, in the end, is a major problem. That is why trans people are often unwilling to engage in public 'debate'. Because the right that liberals so assiduously defend, to intellectualise about issues they only partly understand and that will likely never affect them, can and does end in hurt, emotional and physical, for trans people. In Synestra's case, this debate had very real, very adverse consequences.

CHAPTER 1

Finding Trans

A very ordinary child

When does trans begin? Is it always there, from earliest days? Or is it something one grows into as one gets older? Take a hundred trans adults, and you will hear a hundred different stories. Some just knew, aged four, that there was something not quite right on the gender front. Others achieved self-awareness later – sometimes much later – in their teens, their twenties. In middle age.

There is no single rule of thumb; and then there is the inevitable muddying of the water as individuals look back from later in life, looking for clues. Was that fondness for the dressing-up corner in primary school evidence of future transness? Or nothing more than the natural curiosity and creativity of a child?

What about the tomboy who is never down from the tree in their garden? Or the boy playing about with make-up at 12? These are questions that are asked both ways. Looking forward, parents and specialists wonder whether they are indicators that a child is trans or will turn out to be so. Later in life, individuals look back seeking the first clues of difference.

Synestra's early life provides few hints as to what was to come later. She was born, 16 June 1992, in Grantham Hospital, Bottesford, Nottinghamshire, a few miles west of Grantham. The attending physician declared her a boy; and she was named Alex.

Mum, Amanda, is, like many mothers of trans children,

unexpected warrior and accidental activist. Now a formidable and experienced businesswoman, who campaigns tirelessly for trans children, neither of these things was on the cards when she was younger.

She was born and grew up in Stevenage. At 18, Amanda moved to London where she worked for the next eight years. During that time, she met her future husband through a boyfriend in Spalding. They married quickly, in 1984, and moved out to Hertfordshire, before some three years later moving up to Bottesford. Her partner, an Englishman who had emigrated to South Africa, was a businessman, some ten years her senior. She set up an engineering business, making infrared heat lamps for drying automotive paint for vehicles involved in accident repair. This worked well: her husband was then working for BSAF, a manufacturer of industrial paints, and their business interests dovetailed neatly.

There were ups and downs: at one point the business employed many of the working women as well as half a dozen local welders in Bottesford. But Amanda came a cropper during the 1990/91 recession. She needed additional funding to finance the expansion of her business, but was turned down by her bank. For a while, she managed to carry on by seeking out alternative means of finance. But she over-traded and her business failed.

Every cloud, though, has a silver lining. The experience of having to finance the business, and failing, and then resurrecting it from insolvency taught her about finance. This she put to good use in her second career, which she has pursued for the last 20 years or so, as a finance broker, adviser and consultant to business, mostly small and medium-sized enterprises, but more recently property developers also.

Meanwhile, the couple had been trying for some years to create a family of their own. Her partner already had one daughter from a previous relationship who remained in South Africa. She was 15 when they married, just ten years younger than her new step-mum! For some years they tried for a child and, when this proved unsuccessful, they opted for IVF on many occasions. But the treatment always failed. Eventually Amanda took it upon herself to use donor sperm, and despite doubts as to its effectiveness, it worked first time. Good news! However, Synestra's biological father was unknown and untraceable, and this, as one friend later observed, may in some small way have contributed to later insecurities.

What should have been a happy event proved otherwise. In 1990, Amanda's marriage was struggling, due to her partner's increasing dependence on alcohol. This, in turn, led to behaviour that was both erratic and unreasonable.

Alex/Synestra was just one year old when Amanda decided she could take no more. She moved to a small house in Grantham, and she continued to run her business, and simultaneously care for her child. In 1994, life took a turn for the better. Amanda successfully brought her business back from insolvency and sold it at a profit. In October, she was at a trade show in Bristol, when she met future husband, John De Courcy, also, perhaps inevitably, working in the automotive paint business.

Happy coincidence, or fate: John also hailed from Stevenage. Shortly after, Amanda moved back down to the Stevenage area to be with him. Although Amanda's sister still lived in their birth town, her parents had followed her to the Midlands and were then living in Barkston, a small village on the outskirts of Grantham. The decision to move back was therefore a tough one. On the other hand, staying would put some distance between her and her husband, and it wasn't long before she and John made a new home in the small village of Weston, just north of Stevenage.

John already had two children of his own – Carl, now 38 and Michelle, 39 – living in Ohio, USA. These, together with Adam,

John and Amanda's son, born in 2000, formed the core of the widely dispersed but strong, family within which Alex/Synestra now began to grow up. Carl and Michelle both travelled to the UK and, as a small child, Alex spent many happy days with them. Becky also came to the UK to visit her own family and her father, and until Alex/Syn was six, both were also a regular part of his life. Alex/Syn and Adam attended Carl's wedding (in Ohio). Alex further had a strong and lasting bond with Amanda's mum and dad: the latter survived Syn's death in 2015 by two years.

Alex went to a small village primary school in Weston, a few miles to the north of Stevenage. Early learning difficulties posed a dilemma for teachers, and there were concerns that the continuing influence of Alex's alcoholic father was causing upset and distracting from school work. The latter was keen to maintain a relationship with Alex. However, he and his family were based in Spalding, approximately 80 miles north of where Amanda and Alex were now living.

There were also more serious issues than distance. Amanda's ex was frequently drunk, and Amanda had concerns that he was not fully competent to look after a young child. On one occasion, he picked up Alex and Alex's belongings, and travelled by train to Spalding. He then got off, leaving all his luggage on the train. As a result, they ended up in Spalding with no change of clothes, no nappies, and with Alex's favourite teddy lost in the middle of winter. Returning home, Alex would sometimes talk about bright pills on the fireplace. Coincidence? Or a factor in Synestra's later addiction?

Amanda also discovered that her ex had left Alex, then aged six, in an unlocked flat on a busy street while he went off to buy cigarettes. Concerned for the safety of her child, she and John went to court to try and halt contact. The court refused, ruling that Alex's father was entitled to continuing access.

At this point, the situation was getting to be too much, too stressful. So they took Alex to Malta for the Christmas of 1998, along with Amanda's parents. In the end, it was an unnecessary journey. For Alex's dad was already dead. He died in November of 1998, at the relatively early age of 49, from multiple organ failure caused by chronic alcohol abuse.

Amanda, though, was unaware of this until January 1999, when her mother found out through another friend of the family.

With all of this going on it was difficult to diagnose the root cause of Alex's difficulties at school – and easy to dismiss them as 'just' due to upset over Alex's father. On the plus side, one of the senior teachers at Weston Primary took a personal interest in Alex. She helped the family to obtain a special educational needs diagnosis, including dyslexia, and this brought additional support and lessons at school.

This was the turning point. Everything seemed to click, and Alex, aged eight or nine, took wing. As Amanda puts it, he was 'getting very brilliant at everything'. And while there may be an element of maternal hype to this, his subsequent academic career bears out that he was a very bright child. This was confirmed a couple of years later, when Alex left Weston Primary School, and passed the entry exam into the private, but selective, St Christopher's, Letchworth.

If Alex was gifted academically, he was also outwardly shy. Amanda recalls how, for six years, she would drop Alex off at the gates of his primary school and he would never join in with the boys. Quite the contrary: Amanda remembers him as being always on the sidelines, always not quite part of what was going on. Alex did not make friends easily.

Writing about this period later, Synestra confirms this. She considered herself to have been living a very normal school-life: she did not make friends easily but was looked upon favourably by everyone in her class. Teachers, too, liked her. She was one of those pupils who simply 'got on': she never made enemies and had just one or two close friends throughout her time in primary school, both male.

Also characteristic of Alex at this time were his manners and the trust he clearly had in his parents. One manifestation of this was confidence that parents could be trusted when it came to educating Alex in new tastes. When the family first arrived back in Stevenage, they sent out for a curry. John ordered a chicken korma; Alex tried it and, from then on, was happy to eat curry. In fact, you could take Alex anywhere to eat. A small thing? Perhaps. Though not to any parent who has ever dealt with a fussy eater. As food, so other aspects of Alex's behaviour: he was remarkably accommodating.

Later, as difference emerged in his years at secondary school, Alex/Synestra maintained strong bonds with family and was respectful of parental feelings, even while carving out a unique personal space.

The one exception to Alex's social isolation was a love of swimming and badminton, both sports in which he excelled. These were the only team activities that he willingly joined. Not for him the more traditional boys' team sports, like football or cricket.

Beyond that, Alex's circle was limited to a total of two real friends. Richard and James. Richard, the first to befriend Alex, became a friend in part through circumstance. He lived just around the corner from where the family lived, and John and Amanda were also friends with Richard's parents. So the children saw a lot of one another, often going to the same holiday clubs during the school breaks. James became Alex's best friend around the age of eight.

For a couple of years, these seemed to be all that Alex needed in terms of school friendship. At the same time, this friend deficit was a concern to John and Amanda. The school to which Alex would most likely have gone within the state system had just had a massive extension and, as Amanda understood it, was aiming to increase its pupil roll to 2000.

They worried, with reason, that this would be a disaster. Alex – quiet, subdued – would be swallowed whole by the experience. In the end, Richard opted for this school. James went to another school in Letchworth. And they decided, despite the expense, to send Alex to St Christopher's. This, in hindsight, they consider one of the best decisions they took.

Were there any clues to Syn's gender identity? After all, it is argued by many that transness can and does present early: at age four or five in some cases. Equally, some trans individuals do not come into themselves until later, sometimes much later. It is always tempting to look back through the prism of hindsight for clues. A very common game played by later transitioners is: Was I? Could I have known sooner? or Why didn't I realise sooner? It is a pointless game.

One characteristic of Alex/Synestra that was emerging even then was a tendency to be direct, to the point of rudeness. They didn't like pretending to be someone or something they weren't, and as a result, Alex never got involved in plays. At Christmas, though, in Alex's early days in primary school, he opted to wear a tutu. This was reward, of sorts. The school had 'time-outs', during which the well-behaved children were allowed over to the nursery, where they could pick something to wear from the dressing-up box. Syn's choice of outfit was a pink tutu, which was still being worn at going-home time. As John put it: 'I've gone over there and he's in a bloody dress.' It was, he later said, 'strange, but not worrying'.

Add in the dyslexia, the aloofness, and some of Alex/Syn's early childhood issues. The fact that Syn 'always ran like a girl'! John and Amanda put it down to coordination. Yet if gender identity truly is about modelling oneself on same-gender individuals, perhaps something was there. Perhaps Synestra, as many trans children before her, was hiding it in case it marked her out for adult disapproval.

Or perhaps not. Having never encountered gender dysphoria before, Syn's parents and family put down any eccentricities to the strain of coping with an increasingly erratic non-resident father. Gender issues were nowhere on the radar. In that, they were lucky: they were spared the social disapproval and the sometimes overt discrimination targeted at trans children and their parents that is commonplace in some parts of the UK today.

Transgender kids: the horror!

A few years back, the *Daily Mail* weighed into the debate about transgender children with a snort of outrage about politically correct busybodies pushing a 'transgender agenda' in schools. Or as they put it: 'Schools are labelling children as young as four as "transgender" simply because they want to dress up as the opposite sex.' In that instance, their target was a 2012 Ofsted survey and report, *No Place for Bullying*. I spoke to Ofsted at the time; the aim of this report was to 'evaluate the effectiveness of the actions that schools take to create a positive school culture and to prevent and tackle bullying'. It included guidelines to the effect that if children wished to cross-dress, they should be supported. Or, more precisely, other children should be dissuaded from bullying. Ofsted also set out what they considered to be best practice: '...the culture and ethos in the school were very positive. The schools' expectations and rules clearly spelled out how pupils should interact with each other. Respect for individual differences had a high profile.'

Read the report and it is clear. Ofsted were proposing nothing more revolutionary than talking to pupils and parents, involving them, and ultimately respecting the expression and exploration of difference. Scarcely rocket science!

The basis for this approach is the 2010 Equality Act, which sets out a public duty in respect of any bodies or organisations funded by the state. They must not just deal with discrimination when it arises, but promote positive relations between different groups of people. In other words, there exists a legal mandate to encourage children to be positive about protected characteristics.

One such protected characteristic is 'transgender'. Schools have a responsibility to educate and, more specifically, to work with staff and pupils to eliminate discrimination based on the fact that a child presents as transgender. It is not about finger-wagging and saying no – though that may occasionally be part of the approach. For the most part, though, it is about saying yes to good behaviours that encourage and celebrate diversity.

In respect of gender, if a young child wishes to play with non-standard forms of gender expression, the report proposed no more than that schools give them the space to do so, without being bullied for their pains.

It makes a great deal of sense. If we want a less gendered society, in which all members are equally capable of contributing to the best of their talents, unconstrained by gender expectations, then the less that children are crammed into rigid gender roles, the more likely it is that that will happen. If we want girls to grow up to be scientists and computer programmers, it might help to allow them to dress up as pirates when small. Ditto boys. Or perhaps vice-versa. A few more boy princesses would do no great harm.

In practice, the current received wisdom is to encourage the first – essentially, the masculinising of girls – while discouraging the second, the feminising of boys. This is neither a progressive nor feminist project. Rather, it is simply teaching boys and girls, by means of a pseudo-progressive approach, that being masculine is a good thing, feminine less so.

What works for gender in general terms also works for trans

kids. Or gender-questioning kids. That is just as well, because it is not always clear whether a child is trans or working their way through their ideas about gender. While many trans people can date discovery of their transness back to a very clear point in childhood, not all do. Equally, not every child who questions gender will go on to transition. That, too, is fine. In short, as Ofsted recommended, protect the child, provide support, keep a watchful eye.

Unfortunately, that is not how the media and anti-trans ideologues see it.

Viewing simple kindness as some sort of transgender agenda designed to turn the nation trans, the press has been awash lately with stories designed to sensationalise the issue. 'How can a child know its gender?' is one popular line of attack, conveniently ignoring the fact that the average non-trans child will, indeed, tell you very loudly, very determinedly what his or her gender is from age four onwards.

And if the child does not, its parents certainly will. In autumn 2017, a Christian couple made headlines by threatening to withdraw their child from a class that had just gained a trans child. Their argument: it was wrong and confusing for children, and besides, a child of six was too young to know its gender. 'What gender are *your* children?' was the question put to them on national media: they had two children aged six and eight. Their answer, instant and without reflection was simple: 'They are boys.'

Or, to put it another way, trans children cannot be capable of knowing their gender at age six – but non-trans children can!

Common headline tropes are based on the idea that primary school children are too young to know and – the corollary – that trans children are therefore a construct got up by well-meaning busy-bodies. Or – that transgender agenda again – by a community desperate to increase its numbers through active recruitment.

In October 2016, for instance, journalist Julie Bindel wrote about this issue in the *Daily Mail* under the headline: "'I'm grateful I grew up before children who don't fit stereotypes were assumed to be transgender": Feminist activist Julie Bindel on the danger of playing gender politics with young lives'. Being charitable – assuming that the question is asked in good faith and is not simply an editorial device designed to attack any and all trans affirmative action – that point of view echoes a deeper, more entrenched transphobia. This is the assumption, all too often based on unexamined attitudes in respect of what transness is, that it is somehow linked to sexuality. Therefore it is wrong, impossible, perverse, even.

Sometimes the 'debate' tips over into caricature of itself. The core issue, the nation was informed in early 2017, was whether primary school children ought to undergo gender surgery. No matter that no expert ever suggested such a thing, or that the trans community itself would be aghast at such a suggestion. This was put out not by some tawdry tabloid, with more regard for circulation than the truth. This was tweeted – and then repeated on air – by Emily Maitlis, one of the presenters of the BBC's flagship *Newsnight* programme.

Instant outcry from trans individuals led Maitlis to correct herself. Even then, the correction was only to suggest that the question was about whether primary school children should receive sex-change hormones.

The situation is reinforced by some highly ideological research, which has since given rise to claims that the majority of trans children 'detransition' as puberty approaches. This was given added fuel by a documentary put on by the BBC in January 2017 examining the practices of Ken Zucker and fellow practitioner Ray Blanchard. Many have argued that their approach is tantamount to reparative therapy, a discredited form of treatment that seeks to 'cure' individuals of their transness.

Outwardly, the programme was an examination of 'current issues' in the treatment of trans children. However, many in the trans community objected to the false dichotomy the programme pushed of activists vs scientists. On the one side experts; on the other campaigners. There were also serious concerns as to the potential adverse effects of this programme on trans children.

As a result, the documentary attracted a complaint from a range of trans groups, led by Trans Media Watch, but including Stonewall and LGBT Consortium. However, the complaint was subsequently withdrawn after it became clear that far from discussing issues, the BBC was determined to filter this complaint through a process that salami-sliced issues and dealt with concerns such as child safety on a narrow legalistic basis.

From media debate to trans hate: the slippery slope

A month after the BBC put out this programme, and following a serious attack on a trans child that left her traumatised and unwilling to go to school (Child G, documented in Chapter 2), Susie Green, CEO of Mermaids, which supports parents of transgender children, said: 'Several parents have reported an escalation of abuse and language following the recent negative media coverage. While we cannot be sure that one caused the other, it is a huge coincidence that these incidents closely follow damaging rhetoric that instead of supporting parents of trans children, seeks to undermine and vilify.' She went on: 'It is an incredible shame that children are being targeted in this manner – and the press and the BBC must take responsibility for their role in this.'

Far from being an end to the matter, 2017 was, for most trans people in the UK, a true *annus horribilis*. This was the year when a significant trans backlash surfaced, and it was UK media that led the way. And while media commentators spoke enthusiastically of this being no more than a much-needed debate, the consequences for trans people have frequently been vicious. As a charity that actively supports trans and gender questioning children, Mermaids was at the forefront.

The problem? The 'issue', as the press likes to describe it? This is intimately entwined with a wider moral panic over trans children and the myth, promoted assiduously and, perhaps maliciously, that the trans community is actively recruiting to its ranks. As evidence, critics cite a dramatic rise in demand for trans support services in the UK over the past decade. At the sharp end, medical professionals have spoken of a year-on-year increase in demand for surgery of at least 20% every year for the last few years. However, this is just the end point in a very long process, and there has been a corresponding increase in demand for all support services, from schools to GPs to gender counselling.

There has, indeed, been a rise. The evidence, from generations that transitioned in previous years, is that this is as much a consequence of greater awareness. People know that transition is possible, and about the support services available. At the same time, campaigners for trans rights understand well the appalling consequences of attempting to force transition inappropriately.

Anyone who knows any trans history will be aware of the tragic case of David Reimer. As a boy, David suffered an accident that left his penis damaged and mutilated. He then became victim of an attempt by psychologists and the medical profession to re-assign him as female: to enforce transition. The result: a profoundly unhappy young 'girl' and later, after he detransitioned, a depressed young man who eventually took his own life.

In other words, if any single group of people understand intimately the dangers of inappropriate transition, it is the trans community. They are as horrified by individuals pushed to transition when they should not, as individuals denied the right to transition when they should.

The media campaign kicked off in late 2016 as newspapers reported the story of a mother who lost custody of her child because a court determined that she was 'pushing' the child to transition. The story was complex. Many details have not emerged into the public arena, as confidentiality is deemed to be in the best interests of the child concerned.

This, however, made headlines and kicked off the debate about trans children. Because the trans or gender-questioning status of one child had been called into question, it became open day for debate on the status of all such children.

Earnest opinion pieces, almost exclusively produced by individuals with a known anti-trans agenda, started to appear. The question of whether children could possibly know was very much in the air. So, too, was the darker allegation that the trans community was 'turning' young gay and lesbian children as part of some active recruitment drive.

It was into this feverish environment that the BBC tipped its controversial documentary. The spin-off, in terms of debate and think pieces continued in the months that followed. This increased when the government announced that it was thinking about replacing the current cumbersome and bureaucratic system of gender recognition (the process by which trans individuals change their legally assigned birth gender in the UK) with one based on the principle of self-identification.

That was reflected in a number of serious and worrying trends that, as a journalist, I have become aware of since early 2017. Intimate stories passed to me by parents and young trans people include cases where parents have seen support for their trans/ gender-questioning children from the wider family withdrawn. Parents already embroiled in divorce proceedings, have seen a child's gender status raised as an issue in ongoing custody battles.

This, in turn, raises the concern that whether a child is treated appropriately for gender dysphoria may depend on the whim of a judge with limited to non-existent understanding of gender issues. Worst of all, some parents are now scared to take their child out of the house, for fear of the reaction they might get from some members of the general public.

Unquantifiable, because it is the sort of story unlikely to come my way until some years after the event, is how far this concern has led some parents to push back when their child identifies as 'gender questioning'. Some may now counsel caution, suggesting they wait or, more seriously, simply deny the possibility.

Running in parallel to all of this, as highlighted here and in Chapter 2, has been a step change in the amount and severity of bullying that some children receive. Despite this, the focus of the media debate is on the possibility that in a handful of cases, parents – or children – might have got it wrong: again a caricature of the present situation.

Because, in a population of tens of millions of people, while one can never rule out the possibility that there do exist exceptional cases where a mistake has been made, the continuing emphasis on the risk to a handful of children means that the treatment of many more, who desperately need to be accepted as who they are, is now in question.

Underpinning this wilful refusal to respond to the needs of these children is yet another myth. The press is obsessed with the pushy parent – mother or occasionally father – who has decided to impose transition on their child. Again, this does not survive the most cursory of examinations. Talking to parents of trans children, one theme is constant, consistent: they will support their child through thick and thin, but they wish their child was anything other than trans. They do not reject it. Yet they know that this means that their child will have a much harder life than otherwise.

Despite this, the *Daily Mail* returned to its anti-trans mission in August 2017 with an article headlined 'How 800 children as young as 10 have been given sex change drugs'. That was simply untrue: the drugs involved are not, as the *Mail* colourfully describe them, for the purpose of sex change. They are for stopping puberty. The associated article made this clear, although it still included innuendo that this was all some sort of trans/medical establishment plot to make gender re-assignment more likely.

In addition to describing the drugs as 'controversial' it went on to state that 'powerful monthly hormone injections stop the development of sex organs, breasts, and body hair, making it easier for doctors to carry out sex-swap surgery later'.

Trans Media Watch, an organisation that monitors press coverage of trans issues and, in the most extreme cases, raises problematic pieces with the media concerned, complained. The *Express*, which initially went with a similar headline, backed down. The *Mail* refused, arguing that since the headline was explained in the main article, there was no issue.

The piece included the story of a young trans woman who told how she felt that puberty blockers had saved her life. It also included some quite selective points of view from an anti-LGBT campaigner and a medical professional with a long history of opposing gender transition.

It is of course next to impossible to draw any one-to-one correlation between transphobic abuse and mischievous press coverage. Undoubtedly it plays a part, along with higher media profile in general as well as public figures expressing anti-trans sentiments. US President Donald Trump recently turned explicitly against the trans community, declaring in 2017 that trans people were no longer welcome in the US army. This seems to have enabled a wave of much more explicit transphobic comment on social media – though again, that is next to impossible to prove.

What is not in dispute is the fact that in the month following publication of the *Daily Mail* piece, Mermaids logged a massive increase in online hate directed at them. These specifically cited many of the tropes that had been bubbling up in debate pieces throughout the year. In some instances, they referenced the article itself. Accusations included the suggestion that they were a 'dangerous cult' seeking to 'convert' young people or to 'groom gay kids'. Mermaids CEO Susie Green was even accused of 'chemically castrating' her daughter.

Speaking to the *Guardian* in September 2017, Susie Green revealed that they were now having to block around 20 profiles a day as a result of the abuse they were receiving. This had increased from approximately three a day before publication of the *Daily Mail* piece. Some of this anger was spilling out into the 'real world' with direct (verbal) attacks being made on their organisers when they attended public events such as Manchester Pride.

The result, for trans children, and their parents, is the wholly unnecessary imposition of a battle they shouldn't need to fight: a 'debate' around a series of red herrings put forward by people who have done a little research on the subject, and believe they know a great deal about it.

The irony, of course, is that when it comes to dealing with young trans or gender questioning children, best practice is to do little. Affirm their gender identity, insofar as it is clear that they have a view of their own identity. Give them space to explore in terms of clothes, hair, names. Protect them from bullying. And – an important corollary – give them space to back down. Because just as trans children can become desperate when they feel trapped in a role that is not them, so non-trans children can be trapped by well-meaning adults who, deciding that a child is trans, rapidly go on to dictate what that means for a child, and enforce reverse gender stereotypes on them.

Listen to the child and, unless there are good reasons not to, give them your support. This is not extreme: it is simply kind.

In their early years, trans children face all manner of problems. Most of these can be clearly traced back to the society whose rigid gender roles they are supposed to be learning. Bullying at primary school in respect of gender issues tends to be significantly less than it may later become at secondary school. However, as with the case cited earlier in this chapter of the Christian parents concerned that trans children might 'confuse' their own children, rejection often begins with the bigoted attitudes of other parents.

For instance, in this case, involving a trans parent, rather than a trans child, it is clearly the parental bigotry and school inaction that created a serious issue:

When S was aged five, one of his parents began to transition. The majority of parents in the school accepted this and were supportive. One family, however, took a different view. The mum, who had hitherto been friends with S's parents took to shunning them publicly. She also instructed her own children, one of whom was in the same class as S, not to play with him.

As a direct result, a vicious feud kicked off between S and her children. The school, including the head teacher, declared that they did not support her views, but 'she was entitled to hold them'. S, increasingly unsupported in school and faced with bullying from this woman's children, took matters into his own hands – or fists. By Year 4 he was unhappy and acquiring a reputation as an aggressive and unruly child.

All changed when S was transferred to a school where

the policy was 'zero tolerance for bullying'. From disruptive pupil frequently on the receiving end of disciplinary action, including time-outs and detentions, S transformed, almost overnight, to model pupil.

Meanwhile, despite those well-meaning Ofsted guidelines, it is very hit and miss as to whether a school will respect parent and child wishes as regards gender, will do so half-heartedly, or simply refuse to engage at all. In some instances, school attitudes can tip into active abuse of the children they are supposed to be caring for, as the following case studies highlight:

When J was six, her parents approached her primary school and requested that she be allowed to transition socially: in J's case, little more than permitting her to wear gender-appropriate uniform and respecting her choice of name.

Her school, however, in the south of England, flatly refused. Despite the fact that her mother had changed her name by deed poll (not in fact necessary in law, but good enough for the Passport Office and most banks), they refused to use the name by which she was known outside the school and by friends in her class.

She was picked on regularly by the head teacher, who refused to allow her to wear girls' uniform. He also would not allow her to wear her hair in bunches (boys with long hair had to have it in a pony-tail). She was constantly being kept in at playtime sat outside the head's office. Her life was made miserable.

Her mother later told a researcher she was sure the head was trying to force her daughter out of the school. Eventually, a change in senior management plus pressure from outside agencies resulted in this changing and she was accepted by the school, finally, as J. Yet this simple fact of respecting her identity had not been possible without a long and damaging struggle with the school.

In some cases, schools simply refuse to adapt, and put forward unnecessary issues:

A was a five-year-old, assigned male at birth, attending a primary school in London. She was an only child who identified as a girl. Her parents opposed this and sent her to school with very short hair and the most masculine clothes imaginable: heavy boy's shoes – never trainers or anything that might be viewed as unisex, cargo pants, a stiff checked shirt.

Other parents complained to the class teacher that she was plaiting and braiding the hair of the girl in front of her when they sat on the carpet, 'like all the other girls did'. The head teacher told the class teacher to 'stop him from doing that', so she stopped all the girls from doing that, leading to some girls complaining to their parents that they were being told off.

Parents complained again and the head told the class teacher to restrict A's behaviour – and no one else's. The teacher refused, and subsequently resigned in protest. A complaint she made to the local authority about the head was ignored.

A was occasionally sent by parents to stay with an uncle abroad. He would lay out a skirt for her to wear, and as soon as she put it on he would beat her with a stick. They would wait until the bruises healed – relatively quickly on a five-year-old – before shipping her back to the UK. At school, she would head straight for the classroom dressing-up box and emerge as a princess. Some years later, she was known to be a depressed and troubled 12-year-old, unable to learn and rumoured to be taking drugs.

On other occasions, a major part of the problem lies with schools simply not believing the parent and reinforcing rigid notions of gender. One parent tells of how their son, N, slowly emerged as gender variant from the age of eight. Their school eventually got used to the idea, but the experience was marred, constantly, by issues over loos and individual bullying – by teachers! For instance, the PE teacher would order children to divide by gender – and then very publicly berate N for going with the boys. This, though, is but one story, and it is typical of dozens, hundreds that circulate around the trans community year on year. The idea that trans is a 'done deal' and wholly accepted now within the wider community is just laughable.

Over all, however, is a much greater mistrust, between parents of trans children and those in positions of authority, as underlined by this case from a few short years back:

A mother whose child identified as trans found herself at the centre of an inquisition by social services with, as ultimate risk, the possibility that their children would be taken for permanent adoption.

From the earliest contact, social services – and one social worker in particular – made it plain that they did not understand how a child could be trans. They were provided with the opportunity to talk with experts on the subject, but turned this down.

Then, out of the blue, they turned up one night, with police in tow, broke down the door of the family home and forcibly removed two children from their mother's custody.

In court, lawyers for social services made a number of misleading allegations: they claimed that the family was a flight risk, despite the fact they had only just taken out a 12-month lease on a rented property; they claimed the mother was mentally disturbed and, when a psychiatrist reported back that she was not, demanded a second opinion from a psychiatrist of their choosing. They also demanded the right to be present at all future meetings between gender specialist services and the children, despite the fact that such presence would be distracting and wholly inappropriate.

In the end, the judge gave short shrift to the social services department. The children were returned to their family home. Yet social services continued to probe every detail of the family's life in a manner that was both intrusive and intimidating. Result: the girl is still transitioning – but she has constant nightmares and lives in fear of being separated from her mother. And mum's partner, eventually unable to cope with this constant pressure, regretfully left.

One might imagine it gets better as a child matures: that at some point, at some age, they are presumed to know their own mind. Not so, as one parent discovered to her horror in summer of 2017:

L (name withheld to protect the individuals involved) has a trans daughter, C, aged 25. This girl has always been nervous about social interaction, and this has not been helped by the fact that from the age of 17, she has been transitioning, with full support from NHS gender identity services. The latter – her decision to transition – led to significant bullying, which transformed her anxiety issues into something closer to agoraphobia, with C becoming afraid to leave the house.

L and her daughter decided to seek advice and support from the local mental health support team for this anxiety. What happened next quite took her breath away. No, that is understatement: it left both her and her daughter traumatised. Her daughter is now even more unwilling to leave the 'safety' of her home than previously.

After waiting some 18 months for a first appointment, a care coordinator visited. She had no experience of trans issues and from the outset, according to C, was 'abrupt' and 'pushy'. C's transition was not mentioned. Despite this, the care coordinator returned after her visit with a consent form that would allow her to speak to C's gender clinic. C refused. When she asked why this was needed, the care coordinator explained: 'I want to make sure we are all on the same page.'

In the end, she visited some five times over a space of months. On the last two occasions that she visited, C was left in tears. She said that she felt unsafe and judged. As a result, C spoke very little to the coordinator and, after the last visit, she asked L: 'Mum, please phone and tell her I don't want to continue seeing her.'

That appeared to be the end of that. Four weeks later, L was contacted by police and social workers. An adult safeguarding report had been made, accusing L of forcing C to transition. It included concerns regarding C's 'mental capacity'. It should be noted that apart from the social anxiety there was no prior concern that L's daughter was in any way of diminished mental capacity: she was an adult quite capable of making decisions for herself.

Further, before being accepted as a patient by gender identity services, L's daughter would have undergone screening to eliminate other possible mental health related issues that might underpin any desire to transition.

This, in turn, resulted in two nerve-wracking and traumatic encounters. The police came accompanied by a social worker. Together they spent two hours talking to L and her daughter, while refusing to make clear why they were there. A few days later, social workers came to assess the situation. According to L, despite sky-high anxiety levels, C spoke well both with L present and in a one-to-one session with the social work team. She made clear that she felt 'judged' and scared by the coordinator.

She told them she felt that this coordinator was questioning her authenticity as a woman. She said: 'She obviously just saw me as a man dressed as a woman…she wanted to take away the one support I have had in my life, my mum.'

Both police, and social workers were apologetic, explaining that they had to follow up when a concern was raised. They left happy there was nothing untoward going on. That may seem superficially reasonable. Yet the excuse wears ever thinner. For the experience of the trans community has been of far too many baseless complaints of this type being raised and listened to apparently for the sole reason that one of the individuals in a family situation is trans.

It also turns out that despite being refused permission to contact the gender identity clinic, the care coordinator went ahead and did so, in the process expressing concerns about mental capacity and the possibility that C was being 'pushed' by her mother.

Both L and her daughter lodged formal complaints about the individual who they believe acted maliciously.

Finally, in November 2017, their complaints were upheld by the mental health team, and their experience is now to be used as an example of how NOT to do things. They were lucky. Others who have undergone similar discrimination have found that after working their way through a complex and bureaucratic complaints process, they find only more of the same: social workers closing ranks and insisting, as so often happens, that this was a one-of-a-kind transgression.

Meanwhile, C is as anxious as ever – more anxious – and in L's words, some months after the event: 'Still today, if my door goes at an unusual time, I fill with fear. I don't think this will ever leave my daughter or I.'

These, sadly, are but the tip of the iceberg. At any one time, my journalistic casebook has one or two such stories kicking around. For the most part they remain untold. Either because the individuals concerned are fearful of what might happen if their story becomes public knowledge, or because publication is blocked for some other reason.

In the case of primary school children, there are two reasons why this happens. First, and understandably, press regulations mean that many papers are reluctant to tell stories that involve younger people. This is admirable, since it is an important safeguard against children being exploited by media or even damaged by insensitive publicity.

Less good is a reason all too familiar to journalists: 'story inflation'. That is, events that are initially newsworthy become less so, over time, if they keep on happening. If a child being bullied at school is news this week, it is less likely to be so next week, unless there are aggravating circumstances. Once next week's story becomes the norm, then it is not news unless something even worse takes place.

This, perhaps, explains why, in recent months, the press have been largely uninterested in mistreatment of trans children in school. The only major story to make the press was one in which a trans child was shot at following months of bullying.

Perhaps that is 'just the way it is' when it comes to news reporting. What it does mean is that stories reflecting the real trans experience are mostly untold. Meanwhile, papers focus on abstract debates, which, if they do anything, tend only to exacerbate the problem for trans children.

CHAPTER 2

Coming Out

Teen years

As the move from primary to secondary school came closer, Syn's parents were worried. As Amanda explained: 'We didn't know what to do with Syn. We worried because she was such an insular person. We felt she would be overlooked at the local school, Knights Templar in Baldock. This was also a school about to expand, dramatically, and would soon be "home" to some 1800 young people.'

Luckily for Syn, and for all concerned, Weston is little more than a stone's throw from Letchworth, home to the seriously 'alternative' St Christopher's. Once this was an easy target for caricaturists: a prime example of what happens when you let the liberals have their own way. Letchworth has calmed down a little from its early days as a home for 'cranks' and 'extremists'. Nonetheless, it still nurtures various relics of those earlier, more alternative days, and St Christopher's is one such.

St Christopher's describes itself as 'an independent school for girls and boys aged 3–18', where young people are treated as individuals and encouraged to develop into 'capable, imaginative, responsible people with a zest for life'. Unlike many other secondary establishments, it appears to live up to what it says on the tin.

It is a relatively small school by modern standards – just

600 pupils – and progressive in its outlook. It was initially sponsored by the Theosophical Society, an obscure and eclectic offshoot of the World's religions, sciences and philosophies. The school has no formal uniform; pupils are encouraged to address teachers by their first names; and the diet for boarders and day pupils alike is vegetarian.

The latter, as Amanda wryly observes, was one of the few points of dissent for Synestra. In later years, Syn could never make up her mind what to eat: but, Amanda recalls, 'she always managed to find the best meal on the table' – and, given her lifestyle, she ate in some of the most fabulous places imaginable. For now, however, on returning from school she was no sooner through the door than she would demand: 'Mum, I'm starving, cook me some meat.'

At around £4000 a term, St Christopher's is not cheap – 'reassuringly expensive', as Amanda described it. Even though fees were a major outlay, both John and Amanda determined to afford it as they were sure it was 'absolutely the right place' for her. The ethos of the school certainly seemed to agree with Syn and, as the years went by, had a significant positive effect on her well-being. She started there at age 11, and it was soon clear that this was to be a repeat of the primary years: school liked her – and she enjoyed school.

Academically, Syn oriented rapidly towards maths and the sciences, where she excelled. She was not so good with music or languages. She attempted Spanish and German, but in the end was puzzled as to why anyone would bother. As she put it: 'Why would I want to speak another language?'

Another plus for Syn was that St Christopher's allowed her to opt out of 'gendered sport', which she hated with a passion. Not for her team games like football or rugby. Syn played a couple of games of rugby and did not like it...and that was that! There was no pressure for Syn to join in, no requirement to get into 'masculine games'. That was a massive relief to all concerned and, as Amanda put it later: 'I just cannot imagine how she would have coped anywhere else.'

She went instead for swimming, at which she excelled, and which she loved, as well as badminton and tennis. She played badminton about once a week. She won prizes and medals, many of which can still be seen adorning the walls of her parents' home.

She was less involved in the rich artistic and cultural life that was supported within the school. She also remained limited when it came to friends, swapping one James, her confidant from primary school for another. It was with this second James that she formed a strong one-to-one bond during her time at St Christopher's. In later life, she would mix more widely and build a significant social circle of friends and followers online and in person. For now, at school, she stayed focused on one person at a time.

Despite this, Syn was far from a recluse. She was different, certainly, but different in a way that drew people to her. She loved to be helpful, and nowhere was that helpfulness more apparent than in her relationship with her brother, Adam.

Unlike Syn, Adam never focused on the academic. Rather, his parents freely admit, he is sharp, practical: always much sharper than Syn. He knew where he lived by the age of three; Syn was still getting lost at 20! There was rivalry, and falling-out, as one would expect between siblings. There was also closeness and mutual support.

Syn celebrated her ability to help Adam. As GCSEs loomed on the horizon, it was obvious that learning and revision did not come easily to Adam the way they had for Syn. No problem: Syn would teach him all the tricks. She went through the syllabus, looked at past exam papers and put together a crib sheet based on questions and answers from previous years. This was good, helpful stuff and, as Adam put it, 'Syn makes it fun.' In the end, he passed his GCSEs by the skin of his teeth: a success owed at least in part to Syn's input.

Here is cleverness, as well, perhaps, as a willingness to look for the shortcut: the cunning strategy that would enable her to cut through all the froth. A hint, too, at a strength that later, faced with the interminable bureaucracy of the NHS, would turn to weakness. For this was Syn in her element: picking up a topic, researching, synthesising and feeding it back as a series of helpful actionable answers. This she did and did exceptionally well. What she did not do was deal with pushback, with rejection.

It is equally clear that both at school and in her day-to-day life Syn was motivated by a desire to educate and communicate.

She was an early adopter of alternative lifestyles: by the time she was 13 she was wearing make-up to school and – another plus for St Christopher's – they allowed her to do so. Experiences documented below, as well as in Chapter 1, show that in many schools – almost certainly the majority – challenging the norms of gender expression is dangerous. It frequently attracts resistance if not outright reprisal and punishment.

She 'did the Goth thing': Amanda reckoned that she looked a lot like a younger Ronnie Wood! Syn had rather more contemporary ideas, modelling herself on her Goth heroes, as well as fashion icons and make-up artists such as Jeffree Starr. The aim, as she herself owned later, was androgyne.

She was a fan of Black Sabbath, especially with lights off. She would often be found, sitting in the dark listening to them. She liked hard rock, particularly its European versions, and would listen voraciously to German and Finnish bands.

In her everyday life, she was totally non-violent. At the same time, she had a love–hate relationship with blood and gore, which she lived out through the medium of film and gaming. The latter was her main – her only – outlet for aggression. Like many of her contemporaries, she loved games such as Mortal Kombat, which later played a role in her own personal development.

The only game that appeared to frighten Syn was Alien, based on and closely mirroring the film of the same name. She would arrive in the lounge, where the family were sitting and say: 'Let's put Alien on.' She would hold the game controls until the doors opened, and her character entered the darkened ship where the action took place. Then she would hand the controls over to her father and sit and watch as he played. She was terrified, but she loved being terrified.

Syn first started wearing make-up at around 12 or 13. Initially around the house; she 'loved eyeliner', and here, too, is insight into the essential Syn. For, as she freely acknowledged, she approached every task with a strong sense of perfectionism. Once she decided to use make-up, it was not enough to use it every day: it had to be done right. Absolute perfection was her goal – and that she achieved every single day.

School did not bat an eyelid: if Syn wanted to wear make-up, that was fine by them! And with this green light, Syn increased the scale and extent of her make-up project, adding lipstick to the eyeliner and growing her hair long. There the school did briefly resist. So before getting her way with respect to her hair, Syn experimented, adding highlights when she was 12. She was also a fan of Cyber Dog, a store in the heart of Camden Market selling 'futuristic fashion, rave outfits, and cyber club wear'.

It was about this time, too, that she began to develop an interest in medicine.

At the same time as experimenting with make-up and clothes, Syn was also trying on names for size. Although the school continued to record her attendance as 'Alex' – and her GCSEs were eventually issued in that name – it was clear that she was not happy with it. By her last year she was recognised pretty much universally, by pupils and teachers alike as 'Sphi'.

It was important to her that the name matched who she was.

Some years later, she went through considerable debate, with herself and friends, before adopting Synestra as HER name. Then, though, aged 12 or 13, she tried out a number of name iterations, much as one would try on a new top. Syn loved cats: she was very tactile, rejoicing in the fur and the fluffiness. At one time, the walls of her room were awash with pictures of wild cats. She had, too, a love of soft fluffy toys that stayed with her throughout her life.

So it is perhaps not surprising that her first 'othername' was a cat name. That lasted for a couple of years, until 14 or 15 when Syn went very consciously androgynous...or perhaps agender. Her parents understand that she took on the name 'Sphirex' from a character, or perhaps a friend she knew, in Mortal Kombat. As she explained then, there were two reasons for this choice. First, the character matched her own sense of gender at the time. As well – that slightly arrogant, contrary streak that was to emerge more strongly as the years went by – she liked it because it shortened to 'Sphi', which no one could pronounce.

Despite not participating in the school scene, she was good at art. Amanda's father taught her to draw and she drew pictures for him. Syn also started making a little money from it. One day, an individual simply turned up at their front door and handed over £25 for a painting Syn had done for them. Her parents had not the slightest inkling that this was going on.

One thing led to another. Syn's artistic streak rapidly got tangled up with her make-up skills. One Halloween a young teacher brought her daughter round for Syn to do their make-up. This was the kind of practical application of her skills that Syn loved, and she was brilliant at it.

Yet this was also part of the contradiction at the heart of being Syn. She was a 'loner', but absolutely not a recluse. She was, as many have commented in remembering her, capable of being aloof. Yet she was also attractive, charismatic and very much at the centre of life.

Rather than retire to her room to 'do her own thing', Syn built her network one connection at a time. She had a significant presence on the internet, through Myspace,[1] at a time when others were just about getting used to Facebook. One feature of the internet age, far more than any before, is that unless we consciously erase our past, we cannot help but leave traces behind us as we go, and Syn is still out there, scattered across perhaps a dozen different websites and social media channels.

In this case, the Myspace page is still there: a never to be updated reminder that, aged 13–14, Syn/Sphirex had the insight and intelligence to build an online presence that attracted the best part of 10,000 followers. They were interested in her special mix of Goth/androgyne/music as well as a service that in later years she was providing to followers on YouTube: hints and tips on how to do make-up.

Unlike many other educational establishments, St Christopher's actively celebrated that difference. Her school recognised her as both stable and a good helper to others: pupils went to her, asked for assistance, and she gave it. She was popular – though from a distance, as if a film star or pop icon. Many, it seemed, were in awe of her, and that was partly intellectual – a recognition of her cleverness – and partly recognition of her willingness to stand up and defend herself and her views.

On two notable occasions she got up on stage in front of a school assembly to 'explain herself' to school and fellow pupils. For Syn, it was important to her not just to BE herself, but to bring others into whatever her own understanding of that self might be at the time.

---

1   https://myspace.com/sphirexofficial

The first time was to announce that she might be gay. The second was to defend her religion, after pupils challenged her on this. She described herself as Satanic, though 'pagan' and 'eclectic' might be better labels. From a very young age, she was fascinated with astrology, and would happily expound to anyone who cared to listen about the planets; not just as physical bodies, but the mythical and spiritual aspects of each, too. Stone lore and healing crystals were also a focus for her interest. She explored religions, and along the way she encountered Dennis Wheatley, who wrote extensively about the occult and black magic.

From there it was but a short hop to satanic ritual. However, the absence of this topic in her later conversation and writings suggests that this was at most a passing interest.

It helped that she was a good all-rounder, with a most incredible thirst for knowledge. In 2008, she emerged from GCSEs with five A-stars and five As: one of the highest grade pupils they have ever had. A-levels followed two years later, in 2010. She eventually obtained four, in Maths, Chemistry, Physics and Biology.

If she had a failing, it was what she would later refer to as her 'well-mannered arrogance'. Because cleverness, untempered by wisdom and experience, can very quickly become a barrier between self and other people. Neither John nor Amanda considered themselves to be especially academic and they found it difficult to debate with her. She was, they remember, always very matter of fact. Infuriating too, often concluding an argument with 'Of course it's right. Because that is what it is.'

Never derogatory, always well spoken, and with manners: this was her Achilles heel. She had a brilliance that sometimes got in the way of a deeper understanding of what was at stake. It didn't help that the line between Syn mocking herself, and Syn taking issue with others was always a fine one. John remembers her as having an incredibly wide vocabulary. He said: 'She would use ridiculous words when she felt like it, bury you in a tirade of big words, to the point that you'd not know whether you'd been insulted or not.'

She was 'always right...except when it came to social skills and directions. She couldn't navigate for toffee!'

Academically gifted; still, Syn was very clearly a fully paid-up member of the awkward squad. But she was respected for it.

Unlike in some schools, Syn's reward for challenging convention was not ostracism, but election, by the whole school, to the position of 'General Major Official' to help lead the self-government system in her final year. Amanda is not sure if she put herself forward or was just picked, although, she observes: 'If Syn thought she was most competent for the job, she would have put herself forward – she knew she was clever. She also had a sense of rightness, and if it made sense for her, then she would have done her best to achieve that goal!'

Playing with gender: the view from Synestra

St Christopher's was also where Syn first began to explore her own gender and sex. Writing online some years later, she is clear that her self-perceptions were constantly evolving throughout her teen years before settling down in her early twenties. She recalls her first skirmishes with the gender issue at the age of nine whilst still in primary school.

She was, she writes, in Year 3 or 4 of school when she discovered 'the great fascination that is sex'. A boy, with whom she was friends, in Year 6 and doing sex-ed, provided her with her first explanation of the mechanics of the sexual act, and she was fascinated. She quickly made the journey from fascination to lust and she became enthralled with female anatomy rather than male. However – Synestra is very clear – when it came to fantasising about sexual intimacy she would always, without conscious effort, place herself in the feminine role. She had, she wrote 'no desire to be the wanton boy; rather I craved to be to be the greatly desired girl'.

Like so many teenagers before her, she would stand and look at herself in full-length mirrors, contemplating the adult she would become. As so many trans teenagers before her have done, she was imagining herself not as boy, the gender she was assigned at birth, but as girl. Her deepest wish: to experience life and sex as a woman.

Still, the road to transness is not always straightforward. When Syn was around 12, she became bored with straight porn online. She could not pinpoint the exact moment when she first decided to watch gay porn. Rather, she remembers a general transition. She began by dipping in and out and watching the odd clip, feeling guilty at watching gay porn exclusively. Then, one day, she realised that straight porn bored her: so much so that she felt she was unlikely ever again to have any interest in it.

Unknowingly, Syn was venturing into territory much argued over. All too often, ideology rather than concern for the individual is to the fore. For this is where sexual orientation crosses into, and is confused with, issues of gender identity. It is not hard to see why this might happen.

Where a trans individual assigned male at birth is attracted mostly or exclusively to women, then they are gay or lesbian: they are a woman attracted to women, even if this fact is only explicit post-transition. In a similar way, someone assigned female at birth and attracted mostly or exclusively to men is gay.

What, though, if pre-transition one's interest is in other members of one's assigned gender? Before the public became more generally aware of trans as a thing, the answer seemed obvious: you were gay. Transness, if it entered the equation at all, was little more than a variant of homosexuality. Hence clichés of the limp-wristed homosexual and the butch dyke.

This perspective was reinforced in two ways. The medical

establishment, in the early days of providing support for trans people, frequently demanded 'same-sex attraction'. This was so that, post-transition, the individual would be outwardly heterosexual. The reasoning behind this was complex. It was a toxic mix of homophobia, combined with a medically imposed insistence on 'stealth'. That is, the idea that one could and in some cases should only be allowed to transition if, post-transition one was not detectable as trans.

One reason that trans is so much more in the news nowadays is that the trans community itself has in large part dismantled the insistence on stealth. Many trans individuals are no longer hidden, but out in plain sight.

The second, even more toxic take on the gay/trans debate comes from some sections of feminism, already identified in 'Prelude: Mapping the World of Trans'. The notion that trans ideology is 'stealing' lesbians and gays may be outwardly plausible to people who are neither trans nor gay. The reality, though, as Syn's story suggests, is very different. Individuals may, at certain stages in their lives, be unsure. However, as Syn's later public admission that she is trans makes clear, most people, given time and space to explore their identity, do understand clearly which they are.

For now, though, Syn set out on the road to being gay, as seemed logical to her. Or possibly androgyne. Her father explained later: 'She did not seem to fancy girls – she never had a girlfriend. At age 14, she came out as gay. But the next thing that happened was that she wanted to be androgynous. She asked me: "Why do I have to make a choice about my gender? Why do I have to make a choice about being a man or a woman?" That was when she started to call herself Sphirex. That was possibly part of her confusion about not knowing which path to go down.'

According to Syn: 'The very discovery that gay sex could occur not only enchanted me greatly, but also brought me great comfort as I knew it could allow me to play a receptive role in lovemaking, despite being male. I drew great reassurance from realising my homosexuality and by the time I was 13 I had 'come out' at school with great pride and total confidence in my sexual role and desires.'

She went on: 'I've always had a well-mannered arrogance and an impulsive desire to tell everyone all my quirks. I think it leads to the perception that I'm unable to keep a secret, though really it's just pride coupled with a totally shameless attitude, which is probably derived from great vanity in my own philosophy.'

At 14, as a profusion of online pictures makes clear, Syn became much more focused on her appearance. She began to work out and, to develop a 'good body'. That though is a matter of perspective. As later pictures attest, she was at times quite underweight for her age – a point over which she and her mother did not always see eye to eye. Still, Syn wrote, despite working out and becoming over-muscular for her age she remained entirely submissive in her sexual attitude.

At 15, as already noted, Syn discovered Jeffree Star. This was, perhaps, inevitable. Jeffree Star, some six or seven years Syn's senior, is an American singer-songwriter, make-up artist, fashion designer and model from Orange County, California. A performer, known widely for his transgressive, gender-ambivalent on-stage appearance. Star is a self-described make-up obsessive since the age of 13, with his own line in bold cosmetics created for make-up artists and professionals. He also had a significant presence on Myspace.

Outwardly, this was a match made in heaven. Syn 'quickly became quite infatuated with his appearance'. This also marks a turning point in how Syn viewed her body, as she began to see that make-up could be an alternative means for her to improve her appearance. She started out using her mum's make-up and, she freely admits, was totally incapable. But she set herself the challenge of reproducing what she saw in Jeffree's photos and learned a lot very quickly by trial and error.

The working out continued, but was becoming much less important. Make-up, she felt, was a better way of improving herself as it served a dual role: it allowed her to play a submissive role, and to be pretty. This attachment to submissiveness is alluded to more than once in Syn's writings about herself, as well as in later conversation with friends. It seems to be an important and to some extent overlooked part of her life.

Elsewhere, as already hinted above, there is debate about the blurring of lines between sexual orientation and gender identity. There is an idea, mostly unsubstantiated, that gay and trans are somehow interchangeable. This – Syn's attraction to submission – is, however, something else. It is sometimes thrown at trans people as 'evidence' that being trans is no more than some highly developed sexual fantasy.

But this is a circular argument. It only works if you start from the position that transness is sexual. Whereas if you see trans as something real – a natural variant in gender expression – it no more disproves the validity of trans experience than the fact that some non-trans women are submissive, some dominant, disproves their status as women. From an early age, Syn was agreeable, compliant. She was the sort of child who would do as she was asked without argument. This is who she was. If you are prepared to accept the possibility that those who are trans are socialised, early, to conform to the gender roles of the gender not assigned to them at birth, this makes perfect sense.

Syn's teenage belief that she was gay also makes sense. There are many questions that cannot now be asked. In view of how she later came to identify, it is likely that the gayness was cover for her own passivity and submissiveness, rather than vice-versa.

At the same time, Syn enjoyed playing with other people's

expectations, and that too fits. She was broadly deferential to authority. At the same time, she was constantly looking for places and spaces where she could give vent, safely, to those things she felt set her aside. She 'enjoyed flaunting the slightly shocking juxtaposition of the masculinity of [her] body with the femininity [she] could achieve with make-up on [her] face'.

We have noted already how it was about now that her perfectionism came much more to the fore. As far as she was concerned, if she was to do a thing, she must not just to do it well, but do it perfectly. Some of this may have been for the benefit of others. The sense, though, reading her writings and listening to her talking about her own plans for herself, is that this was for her. It had to be right.

As she grew more confident in what she was doing, she put on make-up for school every day 'without fail...ever!'. Through her time at St Christopher's she would get up early every single day in order to make herself look immaculate. That practice stood her in good stead later, when she was vlogging with make-up tips and techniques to fans seeking to look as fabulous as she did. As she puts it: 'I learnt all my technique and everything I know about application during those senior school years.' By 16, she felt her make-up was of a standard that satisfied even her own perfect ambitions.

There is one slightly awkward footnote to this story of make-up and fabulousness and androgyne that presaged problems to come. At the time, though, it was put down to just 'Syn being Syn'. This was acne, to which Syn was particularly prone, from the age of 14 onward. The make-up was something she did because she enjoyed putting on make-up. It was also about covering up. The issue? Not just the acne, but how Syn handled it as an issue.

She did not tell her parents, at least not at first. She suffered in silence: told no one, until the upset became too much. Then, one evening, she came downstairs, in tears and told Amanda and John she needed to do something about it. That was definitely a thing, all too noticeable in the years that followed: a further working out of Syn's passivity, as well as a barrier to getting help. It took the form of an unwillingness to complain, to make a fuss, to make waves. That may score points in polite society. When it comes to getting support services, often already reluctant to engage with trans people, to help you, it is not a good strategy.

So Syn said nothing until she could stay silent no longer. When she did at last say something, it was clear that she had been doing research behind the scenes. Her parents sent her off to a specialist in Harrow, who placed her on a course of Roaccutane, also known as isotretinoin, a highly effective treatment for severe acne. But she knew, before she arrived, what she needed and, as Amanda observed wryly, she appeared to know more about the drug than 'pretty much every doctor she went to see'.

In Syn's later recollections, though, a cause of serious depression and tears was passed over, with the observation that 'I felt very contented with my appearance aside from acne which I didn't fix with isotretinoin until I was late 17s'.

This is a double whammy. On the one hand, Syn's passive nature meant she was all too willing to suffer in silence. To put up with a situation she found near impossible because to do otherwise was just not her. Adding insult to injury, she knew what she needed. Often she knew well ahead of the experts, and that likely added to her frustration.

Family support

The reaction from Syn's family throughout this period was mixed, but broadly supportive. As far as Amanda was concerned, there was never a time when they did not go along with what Syn was doing: not Adam, nor John, nor John's mother, nor Amanda's parents.

Initially, John struggled with the idea that Syn might be gay. That, in turn, led to relations between John and Syn being more difficult for a while than they might have been.

However, when Syn did finally announce to her family – and the world – that she was transgender and would be seeking to transition, John was wholly supportive. He felt his child was a girl in a boy's body and that, for him, made all the difference. He wanted his girl to flourish and be who she was intended to be. It likely helped that both John and Amanda came from families with a very liberal tradition. John, especially remembers that his own father came from a big family. During the war, stuff was simply shared, without rigid gender rules.

When Syn first began to wear eyeliner and lipstick for school, Amanda was slightly concerned. She was worried less by Syn wearing make-up and more by the possible reaction from school and fellow classmates. When the sky did not cave in, Amanda quickly got used to the idea. She had to as, to begin with, it was her make-up drawer that Syn was raiding!

At that point she started to realise that things were going on on the inside. As yet, though, Syn had said nothing about how she identified. 'Had I known then what I know now I would have spotted it' was Amanda's comment with the benefit of hindsight. Perhaps that applied as much to Syn as to her. For although Syn's family were accepting of what she was doing, and Syn too was living through her own crises of gender and identity, this remained all very passive stuff. Something was happening to Syn: this was not a thing that could be positively engaged with.

This acceptance also had much to do with the fact that no one was hugely surprised. Most close family members felt that as a teenager, Alex had been struggling with 'his' identity. They got that 'something was up', so there was no real backlash and no 'don't agree with trans'.

According to Amanda: 'Even people I expected to have a problem – the older generation, elderly uncles and aunts – were very matter of fact. They didn't understand it, but didn't reject it either. If anything, the response from the older generation was best summed up by her Uncle Ron who joined the rest of the family after bumping into Syn, playing on the PlayStation, aged around 12, and commented, matter-of-factly, 'Alex has make-up on.'

Not everyone got it. John's children, Carl and Michelle knew Syn and her brother Adam. They were frequent visitors from the States, and got on well with Alex. For many years, they kept in touch, but as Alex became first Sphi and then Syn, Carl started to have difficulties. He really did not understand where Syn was headed, or why. In part, that appears to have been reaction to some of the material posted on YouTube which, as will become clearer in Chapter 3, did become much more extreme in the way in which it dealt with sex and sexuality and Syn's views of both. Even in the earlier days, though, Carl was suggesting that Syn's parents should 'stop her putting stuff on'.

Since Syn's death, Carl talks about memories he has of Alex as a boy, rather than Syn as a woman.

Becky, Syn's half sister, was also close to Alex and visited regularly while her father was still alive. Now living in Los Angeles, and married to an American, and with a daughter of her own, she never met Syn and, as Amanda freely admits, she also found it hard to understand. But she was sympathetic, both while Syn was alive and after she died.

It is probably not surprising to find that, in the wider world, the extent to which trans and gender-non-conforming children receive support from their parents impacts significantly on life outcomes. A study in 2012 compared differences in outcomes for a group of young trans people aged 16–24 whose parents were broadly supportive, with those whose parents were not so supportive.

The study[2] was carried out in Canada, but there is no reason to suppose that similar results would not be found in the UK. Of those whose parents were strongly supportive of their gender identity and expression:

- 72% reported being satisfied with their lives (compared with 33% of those with parents who were not strongly supportive)
- 70% reported positive mental health (compared with 15%)
- 66% reported very good or excellent overall health (compared with 31%)
- 23% reported depressive symptoms (compared with 75%)
- 34% reported having contemplated suicide in the past year (compared with 60%), and most tellingly,
- 4% reported having attempted suicide in the past year (compared with 57%).

In a highly personal piece written in 2013, trans journalist and campaigner Paris Lees writes of her own early experiences, of parenting and childhood:

> I was bullied as a child, violently, mercilessly, and constantly. I'm a woman today but back then I was seen as a sissy boy – a fact knocked, kicked and thumped into me at every opportunity when I was too weak to fight back.
>
> 'You're gay', the kids at school would shout, the very worst of insults back then. When shouting wasn't an option they'd write cruel things about me on bits of paper and pass them around the classroom. And when I got home I could

---

2   http://transpulseproject.ca/wp-content/uploads/2012/10/Impacts-of-Strong-Parental-Support-for-Trans-Youth-vFINAL.pdf

expect a clip 'round the earhole for 'talking like a poof'. I wasn't the only victim of your verbal and physical violence.

This piece is a sad, distressing and heartfelt statement of loss and rejection. Instead of protecting Paris from the bullies, her father joined their ranks. His only answer to their mistreatment of Paris was that she should 'man up', stop being a sissy and fight back.

From Paris's perspective, her relationship with her father is no more. Between the lines the hurt is still there for all to read. How parents treat their trans children matters greatly. For if parents won't accept them, the child soon comes to believe that no one else will. And that, once learnt, is a difficult 'truth' to unlearn.

Acceptance – and rejection

Trans teens face much the same issues that gender non-conforming children do before puberty – only more so. There is bullying, which now manifests in more serious, potentially life-threatening ways. There is again the question of whether the school, faced with such problems, will step up to the mark and address them or politely brush them under the carpet.

At this age, the reality of transition is much more real. It is no longer a matter of changing hair styles and first names. Puberty blockers and, later, hormones and even surgery enter the picture. Parents are asked to place greater trust in the judgement of their children and to support them in ways they have not done before. But more of that later.

In one sense, what happens to trans children in their teen years is a replay of what happens when they are at primary school, only more so. Schools and institutions that are good continue to be good. Schools and institutions that are bad get worse. The scale and scope for violence against trans children becomes more severe. Those directly involved, still legally 'children', become that much more active participants in how they are treated. Or at least they should do.

These first two cases highlight the level of violence that trans children regularly face when in secondary school.

E was 13 and attempting to transition in school. She had known she was trans from an early age and, having convinced her parents of this, she had their support.

One day a boy in her class attacked her. He hit her with a bat and stabbed her with a pen. She also had chewing gum put in her hair. This followed months of harassment and bullying, both verbal and physical. The response by the school was to give the boy one hour's detention.

E decided she could no longer go to school, and started school refusing. All the school tried to do was off-roll her. Eventually she received five hours a week of home tuition. She was at home all day and engaging in self-harming and substance abuse at night, sometimes disappearing for days on end. Her parents eventually found out she had been raped by a burglar who broke into her house during the day while she was there alone.

Eventually her parents managed to get her surgery at 19, after which she was calm, lost her self-destructive urges, and stopped substance abuse.

Another case hit the national headlines in February 2017, because it was so extreme.

In that month, parents – and media – were shocked by the story of G, a young trans girl, aged 11, left terrified and shaken after a fellow Year 7 classmate shot her with a BB gun. A BB gun, for those unfamiliar with the terminology, is an air gun designed to fire spherical metal projectiles similar to shot pellets and of approximately the same size. They are not technically a firearm and are unlikely to do major damage to a person, unless they impact soft tissue, such as an eye. In such a case the consequence could be serious.

This was backed up by G's mother, who explained that G was hit on the arm and 'no serious damage was done'. But, 'if the pellet had gone into her face or eyes there is no telling what might have happened'. She added: 'Even though G was not physically injured, she was clearly traumatised by what happened. G has previously had to deal with serious bullying and when I arrived, she was just sat there, rocking, staring. It was awful.'

The shooting followed a five-month history of increasingly violent bullying directed against G for being transgender. According to her mother, again: 'G has been attacked several times. Pupils have thrown water over her, spat at her, and kicked her to the ground. Not a day goes by without her being attacked, insulted or threatened with violence... A Year 10 boy accosted her and said that he was going to take her into the gym and beat her up. He was allowed to do this "because she was a boy not a girl". I reported this to G's school and they investigated, but said they couldn't do anything "because there are no witnesses".'

Just two days before the shooting incident, G's mother was called into school because G was 'distressed'. Another child had scribbled 'tranny' and 'freak' and pictures of penises all over her exercise book. They also wrote 'go and suck your mother'.

Why was this happening to G? Her mother echoes the suggestion in Chapter 1 that media coverage was to blame. She said: 'G went through a lot of bullying when she started her new school, but it calmed down before Christmas (2016). It escalated significantly in January 2017, and that escalation coincided with a lot of negative stuff targeted at trans kids in the newspapers. There was also a BBC documentary (the Zucker documentary referred to in Chapter 1) that many interpreted as saying that trans kids were just "making it up".'

Still, the issues, and the causes go much wider. G's mother also expressed concern that the incident was partly a result of the school failing to take the bullying seriously – another theme to emerge in Chapter 1. What followed gave her little reason to conclude otherwise.

'On the morning that G was shot, they did not contact me immediately. I only found out by accident, because I was due for a meeting at the school to discuss an earlier incident. By the time I got there, they had already taken a statement from G, despite her being visibly in distress, and had not contacted the police.'

Her mother insisted on them contacting the police. Yet despite the executive head making all the right noises, their actions (as opposed to words) suggested they were more concerned with minimising the seriousness of the incident in order to save face, rather than taking any real action to protect her daughter.

The police, too, were unwilling to prosecute. From very early on they took the view that this might best be dealt with by means of a restorative justice order which, G's mother understood, would require the perpetrator to admit what they had done, perhaps apologise and undergo some minimum sanction.

She was less than happy with this. She said: 'This is just brushing the matter under the carpet. What happened was premeditated, serious and involved a firearm. In any other circumstance, the perpetrator of such a crime could expect a significant prison sentence. But instead my daughter could be asked to "forgive and forget". Somehow that is meant to make things all OK.' Such an outcome, she made clear, was 'an absolute travesty of justice'. Since then, matters have not improved.

G returned to school. A little later, the boy who had taken the gun into school for her assailant to use confronted G, stating it was 'her fault' his friend had been expelled. This was despite the fact his friend had shot her! The bullying started again. On one occasion, G retaliated, with the result that *she* was rebuked. Shortly after that, her parents decided the safest thing to do with her was to take her out of school, as she was developing serious mental health issues. She was afraid to leave house because she feared someone might kill her. She stopped trusting other people.

For a period, her parents home educated her. Some months later, they applied to a new school where, they hoped, she might get a fresh start. Some hope: on arrival it turned out that the head teacher at G's previous school had been in touch with the head at the new school and given chapter and verse of G's gender history and other issues. They claimed that they had a duty to do so. However, this seems to have been in blatant contravention of the Equality Act 2010. A complaint is now underway.

Of course, one does not even need to identify as trans in order to be subject to bullying:

Twelve-year-old Reuben de Maid, from Cardiff in the UK, hit the headlines in early 2017 when he appeared on *The*

Ellen Show. Host Ellen DeGeneres praised him for his 'uniqueness' and love of make-up. But on his return to the UK, these positive qualities made him a target for bullies in his school.

He spoke of his experience in a video released by anti-bullying initiative, Anti-Bullying Pro. Speaking of his persecutors, he said: 'They would call me names, tell people lies about me, push me, kick me, do whatever they could.'

The bullying soon became a regular part of his school life, taking place both online and face-to-face. Reuben added: 'It made me feel sad and confused why someone would want to be mean to me when I've done nothing to them.'

In the end, Reuben stood up to those bullying him; but this single incident highlights the dangerous path Synestra was walking at school. For one does not even need to identify as LGBT in order to be on the receiving end of coercive bullying.

A major part of the problem is that far too often schools approach transgender children from the perspective of a false moral equivalence. Their perfectly reasonable request, to be protected from bullying and treated with respect, is not taken seriously. It marks them out, in fact, not as vulnerable and in need of particular protection, but as a nuisance, rocking the boat by not conforming to stereotypical gender norms. The result, as in both of the cases above, is schools attempting to downplay the harm being done to trans children and/or ignoring the bullying until it becomes a major issue. On occasion it gets worse, with the school actively participating in the bullying.

Another story – this from 2012 – is that of Ashlyn River Rose of Boston, Lincolnshire. This made national news headlines. In part, for the bravery displayed by Ashlyn; in part, too, because this story, of a trans teenager toppling establishment bigotry, was just too good to pass up.

Ashlyn understood that she was transgender at the age of 14. Like Synestra, she was lucky. Mostly. Friends and family were positive. Her mother accepted her coming out with an encouraging: 'If that's what you need, you go for it!'

School, the Giles Academy in Old Leake, was less supportive. Ashlyn endured bullying from other pupils. She was beaten and spat at; her school bag was taken from her, its contents emptied across the playground; her locker was smashed in.

However, when she raised this with teachers it became clear very quickly that as far as they were concerned, *she* was the problem. The general attitude, she says, was that she should 'tone it down'.

By now, Ashlyn was receiving treatment through the NHS. Initially, this included therapy and guidance under the auspices of Lincolnshire Child Mental Health Services. Later she attended the Tavistock. Her local therapist, she tells me, offered her school awareness training. He offered to put the head teacher in touch with the head of another local school that had also had to deal with issues arising from having a trans pupil.

But the Giles Academy wasn't interested. This despite the claim, posted on their website, that they are an 'Ofsted Outstanding school in a caring environment with robust Equalities Policies'.

Well, up to a point. According to Ashlyn, again, one teacher received a warning because of her behaviour towards her. In front of other pupils, she mocked how Ashlyn talked, calling her a liar and attention seeker. She also made fun of how Ashlyn walked. The teacher was later subject to the school's internal disciplinary procedures.

Matters got worse when Ashlyn started Year 11, her GCSE year. Until then, what she wore had not been an issue as school uniform was not gendered. In that year, though, boys and girls were required to take on different, 'gender-appropriate' versions of their uniform. Despite living full-time as a girl, Ashlyn says it was made very clear to her that, should she contradict this policy, she would be out. Instantly.

So it went, until Ashlyn's last day. This is where the story made national headlines and catapulted her into brief media stardom.

She arrived at school wearing the appropriate girls' uniform. During lesson time, she was confined to a room with one other student. She was told she was not permitted to go out at break for fear of embarrassing the school. After half term, again wearing the girls' uniform, Ashlyn returned to school to take her Maths exam. She was told that the head teacher, Mr Chris Walls, wished to see her.

Once more, it was made clear to Ashlyn that as far as Mr Walls was concerned, *she* was the problem. She was told she could not take the exam unless she was in the boys' uniform.

This time, though, the tables were turned. Ashlyn had taken the initiative and printed out a copy of the Equality Act 2010, which she laid before the head teacher. Reluctantly, he gave the go-ahead for her to sit her exam; still, she was made to sit apart from other pupils.

Ashlyn went on to study English, Sociology and Communications at her local college. Despite the lack of support from her school she still scored an A* in her English GCSE and five other GCSE A–C grades. Her school, by contrast, remained unrepentant. Responding to the allegations, the school stated: 'Giles Academy is an Ofsted Outstanding school in a caring environment with robust Equalities Policies. The Governing Body of the Academy rejects all the allegations.'

Sometimes, the discrimination is casual, almost reflex. An academic study highlighted the case of a trans girl in southwest London who was just beginning to transition socially. Since she was predicted to do very well in her GCSEs in her state school, she applied to enter the sixth forms of a number of private schools. She applied to four, the first three as a boy and the final one, which was her preference, she applied to as a trans girl.

This one turned her down flat. The other three offered her scholarships.

At least Ashlyn had a supportive mother. That is by no means always the case. In October 2016, a very different story hit the news, when the parents of a 14-year-old girl took legal action challenging their local authority, which was supporting their daughter's right to transition. That is, their child, assigned female at birth, had expressed a desire to transition to male. As the first step in this process, they wished to change their name to a more typically male one.

Their parents, backed by Christian group Christian Concern objected. Here, and in many similar cases backed by this group, the argument is advanced that 'their daughter' was too young to take such a dramatic decision – whereas, in fact, no more is asked than the right to determine for themselves what name they were known by – and that their rights as parents were being eroded. This was because their child had received the support of her local authority who, it was reported, had threatened to take the child into care if the parents continued to thwart their wishes.

This case, too, made national headlines. That, in part, is because it followed shortly after another high-profile case in which a mother lost custody of her seven-year-old child. She wanted to support what she claimed were her child's wishes to transition from boy to girl. Her ex-husband successfully argued in court that this was not so.

The press love 'trends'. In late 2016, the number of cases of parents embarking on legal challenges against bodies that, they considered, had impinged on their rights as parents was in the news. This was especially the case in respect of trans children.

At the time of writing, many of these cases remain unresolved. An additional factor here is the principle of 'Gillick competence'.

This came about after Christian parent, Victoria Gillick, took her local health authority to court. She discovered that a GP had provided contraception to one of her daughters, then aged under 16, without consulting her, the child's mother. At issue: can a child, under 16 years of age, consent to his or her own medical treatment?

The case was argued all the way to the House of Lords. It eventually gave rise to the principle that 'the parental right to determine whether or not their minor child below the age of sixteen will have medical treatment terminates if and when the child achieves sufficient understanding and intelligence to understand fully what is proposed'.

This was irony cubed. An action designed to limit the right of children to take control of their own lives became, instead, the basis for significant emancipation of all children from their parents. That was the precise opposite of what the Christian groups then backing Victoria Gillick intended.

That ruling has had significant impact on the medical treatment of children, both through the establishment of the broad principle of Gillick competence as well as the 'Fraser guidelines', which relate to access by those aged under 16 to contraception. The rebranding in this case appears to owe much to the sentiment that it would be inappropriate for one of the great liberating principles of English law to be named after the individual who sought to prevent the principle from being created in the first place. What effect it may have on access to treatment for individuals who identify as trans has yet to be clarified. However, a sounding-out of legal opinion suggests that in time, trans children too may find themselves benefiting from Gillick competence/Fraser guidelines.

The problem is that how schools deal with the children in their care can have a significant impact on their emotional health and well-being. In extreme cases, it can contribute to serious harm. This seems to have been the case of trans teen, Leo Etherington, who killed himself, aged 15, in May 2017.

According to the coroner's report, a few months later, Leo came out at home and at school, and was known by that name to friends and classmates. However, teachers at Wycombe High School, an all-girls grammar school, told him that he could not change his name on the register for another year. According to the school, he 'had to be 16 to change his name'. This is wrong, both in fact and in law. It also appears to be yet another instance of a school deciding to place petty authority before the well-being of pupils.

To insist a pupil respond to a name they no longer recognise and refuse to be called by is nit-picking. As with all suicides, many factors will have been behind Leo's decision. Yet even in death, the school insisted on having its own way. Head teacher, Sharon Cromie, it is reported, then used his former name in her tribute. 'L...' she pointedly remarked, 'was a wonderful person in every way and is missed by us all.'

Best practice for gender and diversity

What does best practice look like in this respect? One approach, which has been endorsed by independent research is the

Educate and Celebrate programme. Created by Elly Barnes and independently evaluated by Anna Carlile of Goldsmiths, University of London, this was designed to 'usualise LGBT people'. Originally a teacher, Barnes felt that she could do more to promote diversity by working with many schools. She therefore left teaching in order to develop the Educate and Celebrate approach, initially in Durham and Birmingham, including schools for children with special needs, faith schools and schools serving faith communities.

The programme, intended to bring about deep-rooted change within the culture of schools, is based on five pillars:

- *Policy*: The start point is in the policies that schools have for dealing with diversity issues. In the first instance, Barnes goes into schools and reviews existing policies in order to bring them up to date. Thus, in respect of trans children, this might involve rewriting the uniform policy, to reference 'children' in place of 'girls and boys', and making clear that a range of options (perhaps clothing traditionally thought of as gendered) is available to all.

   At the same time, policies are brought into line across all of the protected characteristics listed in the Equality Act. The aim is to make clear that one form of discrimination is not more – or less – serious than any other. Thus, when it comes to use of language, a school might, in the past, have given a child a one-day exclusion for use of racist language, but only a telling-off for transphobic comment. By ensuring that the penalty for using transphobic language is the same as for using racist language, this makes clear in the most practical way possible that neither is tolerated.

- *Curriculum*: At one level, this is about bringing in background material that writes about difference. Thus, at primary school level, books such as *Elmer* or *King and*

King can be used to alert children to the fact of diversity. However, this approach continues across subjects. In the English curriculum, for instance, it may be possible to talk about trans characters in Shakespeare. In IT, discussion of Turing may be used to introduce issues of diverse sexuality.

The key point is that such an approach is not didactic, setting out what children 'must' learn. It simply creates a context in which diversity is normalised.

- *Training*: All school staff are trained in what is and what is not acceptable behaviour and language. In part, this is about setting out a range of acceptable approaches. The aim is to make it less likely that someone will say something stupid or exclusionary about gender-neutral toilets, or about the clothes that an individual child is wearing.
- *Community and environment*: Diversity is brought into school activity at all levels. Examples might include bake-offs with rainbow cakes, singing competitions that include material on LGBT/diversity and rainbow artwork put up in corridors. School notice boards help with this focus by listing out the Equality Act characteristics and making clear what is and what is not acceptable within the school community.
- A *Pride Youth Network*: This is open to young people who identify as LGBTQ or as LGBTQ allies. It is a place where children can talk to one another about issues, come up with solutions, and provide support to one another.

The evidence to date suggests that this generates a genuine sense of diversity. Research from Stonewall and elsewhere is that where such programmes are in place, bullying as a problem dissipates.

A key finding from this report is that once a school has made children feel safe in respect of gender identity and orientation (LGBT) this has a rolling effect, pushing down on other -isms, such as racism. It helps too by removing one of the major barriers to teachers being supportive of equality and diversity programmes, which is fear of failure.

That is, teachers are often very worried about 'getting it wrong'. They are afraid of using the wrong word or pronoun or misunderstanding a particular issue. Rather than try to do the right thing or engage, teachers often 'lock down' when it comes to issues of diversity, restricting themselves to input that is narrow and broadly 'safe' in order to protect themselves from criticism.

One focus of these programmes is teaching that people will make mistakes. However, as long as these were well intentioned, and as long as there is learning and progress, it is no big deal. It is OK to discuss things openly, factually. With pressure off, both teachers and pupils feel freer to experiment and, over time, to improve.

In the early years, particularly in primary school, it is not just about trans. When people talk about trans, they visualise Caitlin Jenner. They don't think of gender non-conforming kids and kids with parents doing non-gender-specific jobs. In one school, for a reading of the book *Boy in a Dress*, a male teacher came in wearing a dress. Several boys followed suit. A teaching assistant involved in that exercise talked about how boys who 'dressed up' focused on female stereotypes. For instance, they tended to produce an exaggerated 'female' or 'drag queen walk'. After this policy was introduced, and space was made for them to discuss their perceptions of women, they shifted to more conventional walking when they dressed up. This is not unusual: when children are introduced to trans issues, there is often a significant halo effect, leading them to rethink their attitudes to LGBT and gender issues more widely.

Again, this fits with what is known about the way in which children – especially boys – respond to diversity initiatives. Playing with political incorrectness – telling racist/sexist/anti-LGBT jokes – is a stage and a part of testing boundaries. The role of parents and teachers of young people between ages of 12 and 18 is not just about setting down rigid rules, but also about keeping lines of communication open. They need to make clear that boundaries exist and that overstepping them is unacceptable.

Research again suggests that the strictest parenting styles tend to produce the most damaged children, either physically or mentally.

Contrary to the cliché to be found in some quarters, such initiatives are not just for liberal/progressive schools in affluent areas. Educate and Celebrate applies equally to secondary schools and to areas traditionally thought of as beyond help.

One project was started in a northern secondary school in an area that would be generally described as deprived. There were few jobs, and a monoculture that was politically anything but liberal. Within the school was a young trans guy, in Year 10. He had been kicked out by his family and was living with a lesbian friend.

The scope for further bullying and ostracism in school was clear. However, the school actively pursued the Educate and Celebrate programme, and this made a difference. According to the teacher in charge of running the Pride Youth Network: 'The lad had come along to football practice as a boy and he passed quite well and the other lads in the football were like: "What do we call them? Is it him?" I told them that of course that was OK, and he is now fully accepted by his (male) peer group.'

Educate and Celebrate is holistic and, once embedded, it works to situate LGBTQ positive stuff across the school. Like all such programmes, it depends very much on the level of support provided: it is most effective when promoted from the very top, from governors and the head teacher; far less so when it starts from or is perceived as being the responsibility of a junior teacher.

Syn, in the end, was lucky to have found a school that did not need such a programme. St Christopher's delivered diversity and inclusion almost by accident, because such values were deeply ingrained in the school DNA. Elsewhere, as the stories here highlight – and bear in mind, these are but the tip of the iceberg – it is unlikely she would have had such an easy ride.

CHAPTER 3

Girls Just Want to Have Fun!

In 2010, Synestra swapped Stevenage for London, where she planned a career in science. Or perhaps where others had plotted a career for her in science. In her GCSE years, teachers had been eager to point her towards maths and science, and there was talk of her becoming a pilot or a doctor.

That, though was really not her, with the result that like many gifted pupils, Syn ended up going to university with little clue what she wanted to do – but attempting to fit in with other people's expectations of her.

The mother of one of her close childhood friends was a qualified chemist at Roche, and this struck a chord. Science, in general, intrigued her, and she was eclectic, successfully linking her interest in stars and planets and religion to a broader vision of world science.

She interviewed for a place at Trinity College, Cambridge, initially to do medical science. She received a conditional offer, which, she later wrote, she 'blew out of the cosmos'. The Cambridge atmosphere, she suspected, perhaps rightly, would have been too stifling for her. Besides it was just down the road from Stevenage, a similar distance to London, but, it seems, the bright lights beckoned.

She was then accepted by University College London for a

place on their Natural Sciences course. No: more than a place, she won a bursary, sponsored by the Sir John Cass's Foundation, which aims to assist brighter students through education. Since the cost of a university place in London is that much higher than elsewhere in the country, the Foundation provides a grant of £7000 a year towards accommodation.

This was one of her prouder moments. Syn attended, with her family, a ceremony that took place during the Lord Mayor's Banquet. She was the only student in her year to receive an award for a science subject.

Except, it was not a good fit for her. Syn had already, through her years at school, begun to build up a large-scale following online – through Myspace initially and later through YouTube and Tumblr – sharing her skills, her expertise and her passion for make-up with other users. She was good at make-up – an acknowledged expert – and, as when she helped her brother with his GCSE revision, she enjoyed sharing that knowledge with others. Whatever she eventually chose to do, some involvement in training was on the cards.

But – that passivity again! – she likely understood that a pure science career was not for her. Her ambition, inspired by early admiration for Jeffree Star, was to set up her own business, developing and marketing cosmetics. But sensing that such a move would be viewed as 'beneath her' – still locked into meeting other people's expectations – she followed the road of least resistance and started her course at UCL.

Discussing this decision later with friends, she intimated that had she had more courage she would have done what she did eventually decide to do: a BSc in Cosmetic Science with the London University of the Arts. It was a three-year course, which she began in autumn of 2011.

That, though, is to run ahead. A significant development in Syn's life at this time was her friendship with Michael, an individual with whom Syn was on the same wavelength and who has, more recently, followed in Syn's footsteps, transitioning and amending her name to Lux.

They had much in common. They were both 'internet celebs' – albeit minor celebs – through their presence on Myspace and later, from about 2006 onward, on YouTube. There they rapidly registered an audience of millions. In the early days, Lux possibly drew a greater following through her regular broadcasts under the label of 'Androgenetics'. Syn and Lux were both known as 'visually interesting'. Both were make-up artists. Both, basically, boys in make-up with pretty pics. What was not to like?

It was in 2006, at the precocious age of 14, too, that Synestra – then still going by the name of Sphirex – first appeared on Lux's radar. For in addition to being known for her online presence, there was a rumour doing the rounds – not true – that Sphi was dating Gaahl, the lead singer for Norwegian Death Metal group Gorgoroth.

The rumour attracted a fair amount of comment amongst the fan base for this 'long-haired, evil-looking man with corpse paint', as one fan site described him. According to friends of Sphi, this was all it was: rumour. Still, it was an early sign of what would later be noted as her charismatic power to attract.

Sphi and Lux first met, face to face, in 2008. Lux was a year older and working in a jewellery shop in Brighton. A mutual friend, Elliott – who has since gone on to a career as a drag queen in Manchester – brought Sphirex in, and it was not a success. Remembering that occasion, Lux says that Sphi had an air of superiority about her and, largely because of that, she did not take to her at all. It probably did not help that they were also occupying very similar fan-spaces online. They therefore saw one another as rivals rather than as potential allies.

They had little contact for the next year, but in 2009 they bumped into one another at a house party in London. Again, mutual friends were the key to bringing them together: this time an artist group. Both enjoyed partying in London. Ironically, in the light of what followed, both were committed to 'no drugs/no alcohol'. They gelled: two odd-ones-out together.

Remembering that encounter, Lux says: 'Sphi was super goth, was wearing baggy black jeans and a Matrix-style leather jacket. She had long straight black hair, and was wearing a muscle rest to show off her shoulders and arms. At the time, she was very into body-building.'

She goes on: 'We sat on the stairs and for the first time spoke to one another as equals, with nothing else to distract us. We talked non-stop for hours: literature, music, make-up, techniques. We shared our YouTube interests. We chatted about shoes!'

They had other things in common, too: childhood issues, interests. Both had had, in different ways, issues with their fathers. As already noted, Syn's dad had difficulty in dealing with the idea that Syn might be gay. This was resolved by time and Syn's own self-realisation that she was trans. But in 2009, it provided another support to their rapidly strengthening friendship.

A cliché, then, but, as morning broke, they parted good friends. More than that: they were, as Amanda put it, 'two halves of one person, absolutely a pair!'

In 2010, Lux was earning a little money, mostly from photography. Early in the year, she decided to move to London to pursue a degree in fashion photography, preferably with the London College of Fashion. In the end, that particular plan did not work out, for reasons that Lux is sure had more to do with some toxic combination of homophobia/transphobia than her own work.

When she arrived for interview, she was questioned as to why she had changed her name – not, at the time, to Lux, but to another variant on her birth name. She was not presenting as female, but she was wearing make-up. As she puts it: 'At the time, I was still confused and hiding stuff.' This, though, was cue for the interviewer to put to her a number of questions on 'whether Michael was becoming a woman'.

She felt very put upon, and it is likely that this shaded her performance in the interview. Whatever the reason, a call came back a week or so later: there was no room in LCF for Lux or her work which, they politely intimated, they did not much like anyway! Her tutors were amazed. Like Synestra, Lux was another talented individual who had already proved herself in the art she was producing. But that was that, and Lux was left still needing to move to London, but without a confirmed college place to go to.

Lux and Syn, then still calling herself Sphi, now got together as result of one of those all too frequent last-minute student arrangements. To begin with, the two of them got together with a mutual friend to go looking for a place to live in London. However, by the time Lux moved up to London, this third friend was no longer persona grata. So Lux and Sphi went looking for a property for two. Initially, that included looking in the East End, around Bethnal Green. That did not end well.

To begin with, they located a two-bedroom flat for £1300 a month, which Lux described as 'totally disgusting'. At the same time, as they walked away from this flat, an individual approached and told them, in menacing fashion: 'In my country you would have your head cut off.' That was that. Syn and Lux agreed there was absolutely no way they would be living in east London. In early July, their luck changed. They got a call about a 'wonderful apartment' on Benwell Road in north London, on the same road as the Arsenal Emirates Stadium.

Syn took one look and said yes, and despite a certain amount of drama in sorting out a deposit, they were in. They moved in in August, and so began what was possibly one of the happiest times in Syn's life, as she got to do what she wanted, when she wanted and, ultimately, was exceedingly well paid for doing so. For Lux, too, these were good times. As she put it later: 'This was the start of the two best years of my life.'

It was very much a time of 'sex, drugs and rock and roll'. Amanda, in hindsight, wonders if this was the point at which Syn's slide to self-destruction might have been averted.

Life in north London started off rather more tamely though. In 2011, Syn was being paid to do a little modelling and some writing: nothing, though, that would make her fortune. A few days after moving in to their north London flat, Syn and Lux went clubbing – their first proper night out at a club in London – and ended up at Shadow Lounge in Soho. This would later be managed by Dani, another individual who would play a significant part in Syn's life.

Dragarazzi, a model and independent photographer who met Sphi on that occasion, tells how she was inspired by the pair's beauty. She says: 'The whole aesthetic: their make-up was perfect. They looked gorgeous, and they had incredible sense of style.' Sphi, in particular, became a photographic muse. 'I just latched on to Sphi. It helped that they were incredibly photogenic.'

But her admiration for Sphi went beyond the superficial: 'Sphi was intelligent, articulate, well-spoken: not something you come across much in night life. So that was different... Sometimes she would assist me with make-up on shoots. It was a very creative relationship.'

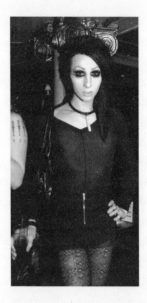 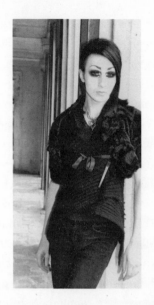

There, too, they met two 'internet gods', according to Lux. These were Mikadoll and Adam Medusa who worked as high-end make-up artists for the Illamasqua cosmetics company. Again, there was that running together of interests in respect of make-up and producing the perfect look, with the fact that these also had a significant online presence, and the four quickly became good friends.

Synestra and Lux were invited to visit the Illamasqua counter in Selfridges. This was a thrill because Illamasqua cater for a very pale look, which fitted well with the Goth image they were both into at the time. In addition to getting to know Mika and Adam, this was their first up close and personal encounter with drag queens such as Jodie Harsh and Dusty O. Soon they were regulars at fashion parties, and while Lux freely admits to feeling a little out of her depth – she has a long-term history of anxiety and depression and when in doubt, tends to back away from new people and new situations – 'nothing ever fazed Syn'. Syn was always the 'strong silent type'.

In early 2012, Syn finally got together with Dani, who was managing a club in Camden called Proud Camden. As with many of the other people Syn was meeting now in London, they had known each other online for around eight years before they met: they shared the same likes, same friends, and Dani was just a year older than Syn.

When Dani first moved to London, a friend invited her to their house for pre-drinks before they went clubbing (in Vauxhall). Dani texted to ask Syn what she was up to. Syn replied that she was available the next day – and Syn turned up wearing 9″ thigh boots and a t-shirt featuring 'an upside-down crucifix filled with kittens'.

This was the start of yet another beautiful friendship!

Meanwhile, Lux was getting work, hosting at clubs. Syn was continuing to model for avant-garde and fashion photographers, including Dragarazzi, writing a little and building up her online presence. Lux remembers fondly the first time all four of them were photographed together: a Rocky Horror Show-style celebration of gender challenge taken at the OMFG club night at the Shadow Lounge. This was the beginning of what she refers to as the genderfuck era: not quite non-stop clubbing, but it felt like it at the time. LGBTQ youth in its finest hours.

There was, too, overlap with an element of the kink community: individuals who liked the gender-variant-with-a-difference girls and boys. Language was problematic: TrannyShack, for instance, was a popular venue, even though many in the more mainstream trans community passionately disliked that name. But they accepted it as just one more feature of the interface between the gay and trans communities.

Meanwhile, Syn and Lux were getting to know one another better, always sparking off one another. Syn was a great fan of multi-media online role-playing games (otherwise known as MMORPG). So was Lux. Both were into World of Warcraft, and they would host gaming all-nighters in their flat.

Amanda later wondered whether she should have put more pressure on Syn to moderate her lifestyle, because this was where she first became acquainted with drugs. Yet even she acknowledged that Syn's time there was blissfully happy. And as far as she is concerned, no blame attaches to Lux. Syn and Lux were total mates, in a way that only two people who like one another and are not in a relationship can be. But at this time there were many influences: people coming and going; and not all, she felt, were good for Syn.

It was a time of laughter and in-jokes and low-level bitching, and opening up. It was not until several days after they had moved in together that either dared take off their make-up. Then it was mutual shock as each saw the other for the first time: without eyebrows, unkempt, unbrushed.

Lux remembers one occasion when she went to the front door to pick up a package, and was greeted by a large, well-muscled delivery guy. He told her: 'I really like your make-up.' No sooner was he done when Syn broke into her impression of him. 'I really like your whore make-up!'

At the same time, for all their closeness, Syn began to strike out on her own. In part because she was the more socially confident. In part because Lux had a body-building boyfriend and Lux was his 'naughty secret'. It is not uncommon in the circles in which Syn and Lux were now travelling, of T-chasers and trans as fetish, for this sort of dynamic to emerge. A great many otherwise 'straight' men enjoy dating trans women, or effeminate guys. Some – though this was not the issue here – are secretly gay.

Lux, though, hated the idea of going out and being a secret. So increasingly, if Syn was going out, Lux would stay in with her boyfriend. She also kept him at arms length from any hint that Syn and Lux were now regular users of drugs and alcohol, as he disapproved of them.

Getting high...

This, though, was the beginning of a problem that was to dominate the remainder of Syn's short life. According to Lux, 'Sphi was still being good girl, doing her course work, and doing well'. At least, she was doing her course work up until the point where she decided to change course and give up on the Natural Science degree at UCL.

In between the studying, of course, there was partying, and very little time to tidy up. The flat 'was a tip', though maybe no worse than many an equivalent student residence.

It was now, though, that drugs started to enter Syn's life, and in fact began to satisfy a wide range of needs that the simplistic 'Just say no' slogan tends to ignore. For the latter positions drug-taking as something wholly irrational and fails to acknowledge that those who do take drugs will often have strong justification, if only to themselves, for their drug-taking.

To begin with, it feels as though drug culture exerted a fascination over Syn. She liked to study things and pull them apart, and drugs were no exception. She had a good grasp of basic biochemistry, and was very capable of dissecting the action and effect of drugs in terms of their chemical impact on her body. For that reason, Syn and Lux both disliked coke: because they understood well that one single amount of coke would change an individual's body chemistry for ever.

For that reason, Lux was not entirely convinced with the final inquest verdict, which stated that there were 'traces of coke in Synestra's system': because when she had been close to Syn, she had been very opposed to using coke.

So Syn spent a lot of her time studying drugs, and occasionally would take performance-enhancing drugs. These served a joint purpose. Her lifestyle was often sleep-poor. So drugs enabled her to spread out the day – and night – and get more done. They helped her to study and do her work.

According to her later commentary, she also seems to have had a certain 'Doors of Perception' thing going on. Taking drugs took her out of the ordinary and into a completely other world of imagination and creativity; and, since she saw herself as able to stay in control, this was a journey that excited her.

To begin with – this was before the UK government clamped down on the range of drugs that could be bought over the counter – legal highs were a major thing for her. B2 was perhaps her first drug of choice, alongside a substance known as Sunshine, which appears to have been either analogue to mephedrone or simply a slang term for mephedrone, aka 'Meow Meow'.

According to Ben, who would later be her boyfriend, Syn claimed that she had been straitlaced until she was 19 or 20 and the first time she ever took drugs was 'with a client'. She was sad, because she felt she would never reach that level of euphoria again.

At this time, Syn focused on drugs with a serotonin-release effect. Serotonin is a neural transmitter sometimes described as one of the body's naturally occurring 'happy chemicals'. It tends to be present when individuals feel significant or important, while serotonin absence or decrease is associated with feelings of loneliness and depression. One effect of mephedrone appears to be to increase serotonin levels. Users report euphoria, stimulation, enhanced appreciation for music, elevated mood, decreased hostility, improved mental function and mild sexual stimulation.

Syn suspected that B2 was also part Meow Meow. However, the consensus in an online forum dedicated to exploring the user impacts of 'recreational' drugs was that it is not.

Overall, the impact of serotonin-release drugs is a little like Ecstasy. Users often snort them, and then – the hippy fantasy – sit around having 'wild conversations about space, time, physics, chemistry'. Syn would spend time sitting upside down on the sofa because that was believed to increase the concentration of the drug to the brain.

Slowly, though, as legal started to become illegal, and one by one, drugs disappeared from the (lawful) marketplace, Syn moved to illegal substances. She started taking etizolam, which may be used to treat insomnia or anxiety attacks. She also took up GHB (gamma hydroxybutyrate), an anaesthetic, often sold as 'Liquid Ecstasy' because of its relaxant and euphoric effects, although it has no relationship to Ecstasy.

Again, the motivation seemed similar to that which went before. GHB reduced inhibition, helped with sleeping, and produced a sensation of mild euphoria and relaxation. It is also used, at times, as a supplement for body-building, and while Syn was now no longer so dedicated to the well-toned body, this may have been an added motivation.

Against this, GHB comes with some significant negatives. It can lead to a loss of body control, with effects similar to alcohol lasting for hours: feeling and being sick, numb muscle and disorientation. More seriously, it is sometimes associated with seizures and collapse, psychosis and severe agitation, tachycardia, delirium, audio and visual hallucinations and paranoia. There is also a strong sexual component associated with the drug's action, which has resulted in it being used as a 'date rape' drug.

GHB can be manufactured with relative ease from a precursor substance known as GBL (gamma butyrolactone), which is typically sold in plastic bottles, often unmarked.

Unsurprisingly, given her chemical skills, Syn started to make her own GHB. She talked about buying the GBL in bulk so that she could process it herself into GHB, though Lux believes she eventually saw that as redundant. By early 2015, Syn had begun dosing herself with lower quantities of raw GBL; once in the body, GBL quickly converts to GHB and produces equivalent effects.

Overdosing on these drugs – GBL and GBH – is all too easy. They are usually sold mixed with water: doses are measured in small quantities, and dosage strength may vary significantly from bottle to bottle. Yet the difference between a recreational dose and overdose may be a matter of millilitres; and for both GHB and GBL the consequences of overdose are dangerous, and include nausea and vomiting, and seizures. In extreme case, overdose can result in coma and respiratory collapse.

All of these substances – GHB, GBL, mephedrone and its analogues – are Class C drugs under the Misuse of Drugs Act 1971. GHB was classified as such in 2003 and GBL, when it became clear that dealers were switching to this as a legal alternative to GHB, in 2009. Mephedrone/'Meow Meow' was declared illegal in 2010. It is against the law to possess them or to sell them for human ingestion.

On the surface, this was all about drugs being used for recreational purposes with a better than average understanding of the pros and cons of each. Unsurprisingly, given that both were interested in the chemistry of drugs and their biochemical impact on the body, Lux and Syn both read widely on how drugs were made, their chemical composition and their impact on neural pathways.

But there is another darker side to the drug-taking, part speculation, part based on commentary from Syn herself. And that is their interplay with the escorting, or sex work, that Syn was increasingly getting into. Because while the front that Syn put on was that this was simply another carefree activity – a means to earn a little money while enjoying herself – there is also some evidence that this pushed her to use more drugs and more extreme versions of the ones she had already tried.

There are various reasons why this may be the case. The scene she was circulating in initially, gay, promiscuous, hedonistic, had close ties to the culture of 'chemsex', the practice of using drugs that enhance sex and decrease inhibition. Commonly used chemsex substances are GHB, mephedrone and 'crystal meth', aka crystal methamphetamine. And while all drugs have a mix of positive and negative association, crystal meth is a step change from what Syn had been doing before. On the plus side, it produces an intense high, accompanied by feelings of self-confidence and motivation. As negative, it is highly addictive, and can lead to over-confidence and feelings of paranoia.

Sex work led Syn to experiment with crystal meth, which, given her already high sense of self-confidence, was not a good choice; also, it seems likely this later led to her developing some symptoms of paranoia.

So drugs were part of the scene she was circulating in: the club scene, where gay met trans. However, in talking with Amanda, there are also suggestions that they were part of the price for remaining within that scene. Syn talked of parties she attended, where the expectation was that she would join in the drug fun. Perhaps that is natural, since just as all the world is suspicious of the single sober person on a pub crawl, so there is a tendency to require all those involved in a chemsex party to be sharing substances.

Darker still, there is some suggestion that there were times when drug-taking was necessary. For despite the happy-go-lucky facade, Syn did not always enjoy her work. Sometimes she needed drugs to get her through.

Whatever the reasoning, what started out as fun experimentation became a significant addiction and, as the inquest later found, a major factor in Syn's death. Lux, sadly, recalls last seeing Syn on her birthday, in June 2015. At the time, she told her to stop – but it seems that warning was too little, too late, as a month later Syn would be dead and drugs would be implicated as a factor in her death.

...and going low

In March of 2011, Syn owned up to Lux that she was getting paid for sex work. It was, Lux remembers, on the night bus on their way home. Syn had left UCL and it was freezing; and at the time, it had not occurred to Lux that without college Syn had no money coming in for rent. Or that without rent she would have to leave London. In the eyes of Syn, who was in all things essentially a creature of logic, the solution was simple.

She enjoyed sex, greatly. She could earn as much as £850 a night through sex work; and she needed the money. Sex work may not have been her ideal solution, but the answer was obvious. And once begun, there was a compelling logic to continuing. Lux and Syn both had expensive make-up and shoe habits. Both enjoyed a wide range of recreational drugs, and sex helped pay for all of these.

In time, too, Syn would start to take hormones. Later still, she would embark on a seriously expensive surgical journey, re-shaping her body to her own very high standards. For that, too, sex would pay: indeed, would have to pay because short of winning the lottery or landing a high-paid job in the City, there was little that came close to fitting the bill.

As Syn put it later: 'I am adequately (intensely to say the least) passionate about changing my gender that I have decided to be brave and become a sex-worker where I have been able to fund my surgeries which will allow me to live happily as a woman.'

The view from planet Syn

Throughout this time and in the two years that followed, three themes – sex, drugs and gender – came to dominate Syn's life. It is tempting to separate these out, to suggest that 'if only Syn had managed to stay clear of the drugs', all would have been well. There is some truth in that. There is no inevitability that being trans would lead, should lead, to sex work or taking drugs. Yet in Syn's case the three came as a package, each supporting and reinforcing the others.

Lux moved out from the north London flat in June/July 2012, when her mother passed away. Syn left a couple of months later, in August 2012. For a month or so, she moved back in with her parents in Stevenage, but shortly after that, she was back in London, moving into her next base, in Lewisham.

From one perspective, those Arsenal years, from 2010 to 2012, were halcyon days: a time of fun and laughter and friendship. They were a time out, perhaps, from being the dutiful daughter that Syn had hitherto seemed to be becoming. Yet it was in north London that she discovered sex and sex work and drugs, which would have such a damaging effect on the rest of her life. Here, as we shall see below, she realised properly that she was trans and set out on an even more difficult journey than the one she had undertaken before.

Here, too, the darker consequences of some of her life choices first began to make themselves felt. A little after the New Year 2012, Syn was raped. Lux remembers the horror of it.

She and Syn started the day as usual, with a minor fashion crisis: Syn had just had a 'terrible haircut' so she accompanied her to a hairdresser to fit extensions. Then they went their separate ways, to two different events. Lux went out with some new friends. In hindsight she wishes she had chosen differently.

At the end of her evening, Syn returned to the flat, and despite the cold she was barefoot. Getting off the tube at Holloway station, she took a slightly circuitous backstreet route to avoid an all-night club where she and Lux had been harassed. But her path crossed that of a man she had never met before, and he proceeded to rape her.

He also stole her phone, her money and her keys. It was around four in the morning. She was out on the street, freezing, with no way to call for help and no way to get into her flat. Luckily, the next-door neighbours invited her in, gave her something to drink and looked after her.

This, Lux felt sure, was a part of what led Syn increasingly to distrust officials. Not just the rape, but the response from the legal system after. Initially she was unwilling to go to the police. This was, after all, 'the sort of stuff that happens to people like me'.

She had a point. Friends persuaded her that if her assailant was found guilty, she would be entitled to several thousand pounds in compensation. This would go some way to helping pay for the surgeries she wanted. So with a little persuasion she took the matter to the police and eventually it wound up in court.

Her attacker was found not guilty, although – Lux's recollection – he may have been found guilty of theft. But in court there was deemed insufficient proof that the sex was not consensual. So that was that. All that could be proven was that he had stolen her phone. Again, friends at the time sensed that Syn felt quite defeated by how difficult and unhelpful the police were. But alongside that was the fact she never spoke about it: and while she railed against other things she considered wrong or unjust this was just the sort of thing that happened to a trans sex worker. Nothing to write home about. Or rather, nothing to write about.

This, together with the passivity already noted, is yet another Syn contradiction: in some things, so assertive and so sure of what she wanted; in others, not wanting to make a fuss. Preferring to sweep even quite serious events under the carpet rather than expose herself in public.

Getting real about gender

In parallel with these events, Syn's view of her gender, which is always at the heart of this, was evolving rapidly. Writing later, Syn was clear that from the age of 15 to 19 – from approximately 2007 to 2012 – she saw herself as a gay male. Her appearance was not dictated by any desire to be an anatomical female. She was happy to be male and had no intention to transition: or perhaps, more accurately, she resisted the temptation to do so.

In 2011/2, however, she began to involve herself with websites aimed at transsexuals and their admirers. Often referred to as 'T-chasers', these are individuals, almost exclusively men, who have a sexual interest in trans women. Or rather, for the most part, they have an interest in transitioning trans women – 'shemales' and 'chicks with dicks'. This interest tends to wane as individuals transition, and their body starts to conform more closely to what might be expected of a non-trans woman.

Syn quickly discovered a new-found popularity, which went well beyond what was there already, based on intrigue or admiration for her appearance. It was massive, beyond anything she had previously imagined, and it was 'totally sexual'. She spent more time in the company of London trans people and eventually, she writes, 'the negative associations with being TS completely evaporated'.

This experience – the confusion of sexuality (whom one is attracted to) with gender identity (the sex one identifies as) – is more common than many realise and is likely related to a lack of information.

Syn dug deep and hit back. She posted: 'So many like myself had spent years resisting the notion that they were a tranny.' She wrote of how energy-draining it was recalling the endless explanations she had had to give that she was 'just a boy in make-up as opposed to a transgendered person'. She spoke, too, of how the constant requirement to justify herself – gay or trans – made her resentful. For rather than allowing her to choose for herself, many gay friends pressured her *not* to transition: not to 'be a tranny'.

One individual, for instance, posted on her blog to say how much they regretted having had 'bottom surgery'. They ended with a warning that there is no turning back, advised Syn not to do it because 'all the guys that used to hit me up no longer do because I just have a synthetic vagina'.

Syn dealt with that one in typical Syn fashion, expressing sympathy, but otherwise dismissing the poster as 'incredibly ignorant'. Some transsexuals actually truly want to be girls, she told them. Clearly you have a lack of empathy for such people. She went on: 'You do not know what goes on in my head and you shouldn't need to be able to accept that SRS is the right thing for me. We may both be trans, but that does not mean that the way you think is the same as the way I do. No two men or women are mentally identical, so why you would assume all M2F transsexuals are baffles me.'

Besides, her previous reticence to identify as trans had far less to do with genitals, far more to do with her ability to continue looking fabulous, which, as many have observed, was important to her. As was her usual approach to any topic, she had spent time studying the ins and outs of hormones and surgery, and in the end, she admits, what convinced her were the possibilities inherent in facial feminisation. Once she understood that she could transition without ending up looking like a 'tragic tranny', the last barriers to going forward were gone.

Precisely when the decision to transition occurred is something we shall never know: the time-line is confused, with subtle differences between Syn's account of her decision and Lux's remembering of it. Lux suspects that the decision was made long before Syn told her.

Photographer Dragarazzi mentions that she last saw Syn in a club in December 2012: it was at Club Anti-Christ for an event called Not New Years Eve. Syn was wearing 'a wonderful white fur coat and the most incredible shoes'. She was 'very girly' and in Dragarazzi's view 'at that point was definitely transitioning'.

Dani concurs, pushing the start date for her transitioning back to even earlier in 2012.

To begin with, though, Lux and Syn presented not as trans but as androgynous individuals who 'didn't want to grow into men'. They medicated testosterone away and did this by ordering an anti-androgen – spironolactone ('spiro') – from the internet. There is a downside to this approach. Quite apart from the cost, which Syn later estimated as sometimes £500 per month, there was no checking the purity of the substance delivered. Or whether, in fact, the substance being delivered was even what it claimed to be.

Many trans women unable to get accepted by the NHS, or who can no longer stomach the seemingly endless NHS waiting lists, choose this route. But it is a dangerous one. A further downside to prolonged use of spiro, or indeed any anti-androgen, is that over time it tends to reduce libido and ability to perform (i.e. no erections). This, though, was less of an issue for Syn, or her clients. She was submissive and beautiful and young and continued to attract an enthusiastic following. At the same time, her libido was rooted in feeling 'unbelievably desirable' to clients and potential lovers. As long as they wanted her, she was happy.

Writing of her decision to begin taking spiro daily, Syn explained that her motive was straightforward. She wanted to stop the further masculinising of her body. She had never had much facial hair; but she was aware that once she'd turned 19, facial and body hair would soon become a greater obstacle to her attempts to maintain her feminine appearance.

There is some discrepancy between her account of her sex work and Lux's. According to Syn, she began escorting shortly after she turned 19 – shortly after June 2011 and not March – though she is clear that it was the promise of abundant cash that won her over.

She talks in a tone at times over-awed of the vast numbers

of men 'totally infatuated with transsexuals'. For the first time – late 2011, perhaps 2012 – the majority of her sexual partners were straight-identified men. Until that point, her relationships and sexual experiences had been for the most part with bisexual and homosexual boys. With this switch, she found herself treated much more like a girl and she did not just enjoy it: she adored it.

As she put it: 'I had been immersed into a world where I was like a goddess and I adored every waking moment where I could experience the unrelenting love from more males than I ever realised was possible. Even the small things about being treated as a girl, like being referred to with a female pronoun, really had me spellbound and still I derive some fleeting moment of pleasure when people naturally go to use she/her etc. in reference to me.'

No doubt those wedded to a more pejorative explanation of transness will translate this into a theory explaining Syn's decision as wholly motivated by sex. That though, is a complete misreading of the situation. This elation during the early stages of transition is common. For many trans individuals, men and women, it represents absolute relief that finally they have been acknowledged to be the gender they know themselves to be. In addition to the actual effects of the hormones, they are buoyed up by knowing they are in the system and, as important, that their body is now very slowly changing.

That someone who works in the sex industry should translate those feelings to a more eroticised context is not remotely surprising, any more than similar comments I have heard from non-trans sex workers who have successfully changed their appearance, either through diet or surgery. This is what people – trans and non-trans alike – tend to do.

In addition to the spiro, Syn started taking hormones – some form of oestrogen, again purchased via the internet – in January 2012. Writing some six months later, shortly before her 20th birthday, she talks of how her transition has brought her 'happiness beyond belief'. Overall, she was in markedly higher spirits. Her life, already 'amazing' before hormones, had now been elevated to 'simply breath-taking'.

Ironically, though, in light of what came next, she also revealed to the world how she was taking steps to formalise her hormone therapy with her GP and psychiatrist. However, as Chapter 4 reveals, that was far easier said than done.

From Synestra's blog:

So yesterday I told my Mum I am Sexually Transitioning, and this was her reply:

"Darling, I know you're happy and I'm really happy for you. I just want you to be happy full stop."...

"I agree that you should have a gender change because you are definitely more girl than boy and you have to live the rest of your life in the right body. Boob job is the easy bit hon, been there, done that! Not sure about the other 'bits' though!! Perhaps you'll make the time to explain it to me as it must be very complicated."...

"Anyway, I always wanted a girl. What you going to call yourself then? Love you xxx"

Alongside this beginning with hormones was another step, which may, for some, feel minor by comparison. But, as anyone who knows trans people will be aware, is often a major shift psychologically. This was Syn's decision to amend her name in line with her new sense of gender. In December 2012, she appears to have formalised this by obtaining a deed poll asserting her new identity. A deed poll is unnecessary, for legal purposes, but is nonetheless a significant psychological marker.

In late 2011, or perhaps early 2012, she announced to the world that henceforth she was to be known as Synestra – or Syn for short – though for the time being she would hold on to Sphirex for the internet.

One online fan asked why she couldn't just stick to Alex and just be Alexandria or Alexandra. Syn explained that she had no attachment to her former boy name, and had not used it for years. In opting to become Synestra she was opting for a name that represented her better and – her love for obscurity – because she wanted a rare name.

If the point of a name is to distinguish and identify an individual, she could not understand why so many people had the same first names: if she had a child, she would pick a truly unusual name for them so that they would avoid being subject to any of the preconceptions associated with a more commonplace name.

A little later, Syn also began posting as Sable Heart. This, she explained was her 'porn star name', as well as the name she continued to keep for escort work. Her real name, though, would be kept for real life. A minor detail; but perhaps a hint that she did recognise that the life she was living at the time as a departure from the norm and that a day would come when she would return to 'reality'.

Syn at large

Syn had amassed a large audience of regular followers: 16,000 subscribers on YouTube and many more on Tumblr. These were certainly not shy of telling her what they thought. And nor was Syn slow in responding: reading her answers one catches glimpses of the self-assurance and self-confidence frequently remarked on by others. At times, though, her reactions shade into a most unmannered arrogance, raising questions of how far this was her, how much the drugs talking.

Though a cautionary note is supplied by long-term friend Dani: 'Beware. Syn wrote within a persona in order to emphasise a character she had created within her writing. So not everything Syn writes should be taken at face value.' Despite this, much of Syn's writing appears to mirror, quite closely, what others have said about her, so that is helpful.

In respect of the sex and drugs, a number of Syn's fans were not happy. As one outraged former fan put it: 'I can understand how people are led into the sex trade & drugs due to desperation and life situations, but actually romanticising it and saying that it is good, that is disgusting.'

Another posted on Syn's Tumblr account:

I feel like my idol just died, I had looked up too you for so long with YT and all then disappearing for personal reasons.. Then coming back [...] I was crushed over what I found.. drugs, proud prostitute.. I know by reading you most likely don't give a shit.. I just want to go back to bed, I don't know if I'd sad for your sake or angry at myself for being stupid looking up to someone who turns out to be like you. [*sic*]

Syn was typically dismissive. She wrote:

You don't know anything about drugs or being a prostitute. Your opinions are so shallow that I can see they have been formed by society and with no measure of personal experience or opinion. You have a lot to learn about life, but unfortunately you shall never learn anything with such an attitude.

Do not be sad for me. I promise, I am happier than you are, and that's all that life is about.

Online, she gave as good as she got. In response to a more matter-of-fact enquiry as to why she used drugs and what drugs she had used, she waxes lyrical. She says:

Most drugs. I cannot explain to you why if you have not tried high doses of uppers. They show you the capacities of your brain. The highest capacity for my brain to comprehend success and happiness/elation. The highest capacity that my brain can experience love. With chemicals I have shown myself my human boundaries, transcending so far out of normal emotional boundaries that one can become apathetic. What stops you? I have also seen the limits of my brain to feel bad and that is a scarier place than you can ever imagine.

Romance and that infamous Syn arrogance. Here she is explaining why people with expertise in science and biology are safer drug-users than the wider population:

I am not entirely against society brainwashing kids into thinking drugs are bad. It has its pros and cons. It definitely saves thick and naive people from starting to use drugs and getting out of their depth, lacking understanding and ruining their lives.

It also makes people very ignorant about drugs, so if you do ever get introduced, you will feel as though everything you have ever been told was so biased that you no longer believe any of it and you will have no tools (unless an enthusiastic chemist/biologist) to use drugs safely to enhance your life.

She has a point – it is a point made, frequently enough, by those working with drug users: that a simplistic 'Just say no' message can do more harm than good. Though here, the reference to those with expertise like her own seems rather more like special pleading: she knew what she was doing and nothing could harm her.

In response to a less hostile challenge, she explained more fully, that she saw cosmetic science, and not prostitution as her career path. But she actually loved escorting, had met some lovely people doing it and, she reckoned, even if she won the lottery would still carry on with it. Ever practical, though, she pointed out that the job paid 'extremely well vs the hours put in', which is great if you are a student!

Mentally, emotionally, she found her work 'empowering and very exciting'. She enjoyed sex, being not the least shy at revealing her personal preferences: 'rough, up against a wall', with maybe the odd hair yank if they require a passionate kiss. If she couldn't do high fashion she would be a porn star!

And, writing a year or so later: she absolutely did not want a monogamous relationship, because that 'only ends in heart-ache'. She wasn't ready for an exclusive relationship: was too young for one. She was looking for open relationships in which she could love without cutting herself off from others. She was still exploring and, she felt, would not be ready to settle down for a few years – at least not until her late twenties – by which time she would have the experience to make an informed choice about who she should be with.

Her responses broadly reflected what was thrown at her. Ask a respectful question and get a respectful answer. Attack her, her choices, as one poster did, and you had better watch out. Here is Syn in full flow:

Society has told you to hold prostitutes and people who take drugs in low regard. You are too young, or too thick, to think for yourself. You will forever be as naive as those before you...the kind of people who condemned blacks to slavery, the kind of people who burned witches at the stake and the kind of IGNORANCE that deemed torture for confession as acceptable, valid and morally justified practices. You cannot use your own brain and make decisions, you merely regurgitate things elders have told you and think that means you have a set of moral beliefs. They are not even your beliefs...you have not assimilated anything...have you tried drugs, do you understand why people take them? Do you even understand why I am an escort?

Set a good example! Have some self-respect! Be a role model for LGBT youth who look up to you. That was never going to go down well with someone who clearly enjoyed their lifestyle choices. Syn stuck up for herself. Above all, she stuck up for her parents. Responding to another who claimed to feel bad for her parents Syn came up with the near perfect answer:

> If my daughter was anything... I would love them. My parents worry too much about me, but they are better parents than you can ever hope to be. Putting your own embarrassment in front of the love of your child.
>
> My parents do not support me being a prostitute, they do not support me taking drugs, but my parents do support me, through thick and thin.
>
> I view myself, less of a daughter to be ashamed of and more of a daughter to be phenomenally proud of.

Transition mechanics
Puberty
Puberty is a time of particular horror for trans teens. From a non-trans perspective, there is some basic appreciation that it is a difficult time when hormones run high and individuals do things they may later regret. However, if your problem is that your body fails to fit your own expectations, then forcing a 'normal' puberty on an individual is not only cruel – but painful and expensive, too.

For young trans people, puberty is often the point at which difference starts to become real – and serious decisions need to be taken. In Syn's case, transition started post-puberty and that almost certainly contributed to some of the issues that she later faced. This is because puberty brings with it a mix of changes to the body as well as the development of secondary sexual characteristics. Some of these may be reversed with relative ease. Others, though, are much more fundamental and require significantly more effort – and expense – to reverse.

For instance, in most cases, a trans woman, taking oestrogen, will develop breasts. These will probably not be on quite the same scale as a non-trans woman of similar physique and ancestry, but they are breasts nonetheless. Trans men will find their voice breaking to the point that it is indistinguishable from a non-trans masculine voice.

But this is not the case when it comes to skeletal changes wrought by puberty. In many ways, the adult woman is simply a larger child. As men go through puberty they undergo a number of changes to their skeleto-muscular configuration – chin, nose, forehead, and, ultimately, vocal chords, which will affect vocal pitch. Women do not undergo similar, or even opposite changes.

A trans woman who has undergone a full male puberty is therefore always more likely to have difficulty passing. If she wishes to 'fit in' as a woman, she may have to undergo extensive and expensive surgery. Facial feminisation, an attempt to return to what their face would have looked like without puberty involves extensive work to some or all of nose, chin, brow.

Voice, once broken, cannot be unbroken. Trans women can undergo training to bring their pitch back from male to an acceptable female range. Alternatively, there exists a procedure – highly risky and therefore one that few trans women choose to undergo – of shortening the vocal chords. The reason for low take-up is that of all surgical procedures, this is possibly the one most likely to go wrong. It is far more risky than genital surgery, with potentially disastrous results for the individual.

Where an individual is diagnosed as trans or identified as likely to be such, but is still considered too young – or lacking the mental competence to commit to the permanent changes that may be initiated by hormone therapy – puberty blockers may be prescribed to halt the development of the undesired secondary sex characteristics of their assigned sex.

These are now commonplace in a number of hospitals and gender clinics across the United States and in the Netherlands, and are increasingly gaining currency in the UK. They allow an adolescent the time to decide whether they genuinely want to go on to transition and are generally considered to be fully reversible. That is, any individual who has second thoughts about transitioning can discontinue blockers at any time and resume their original puberty.

The current protocols for the administration of puberty blockers in the UK are that they may be administered before age 16. However, they are not given lightly. Before puberty blockers are administered, individuals must satisfy stringent criteria that align both to World Professional Association for Transgender Health guidelines as well as to additional guidelines put in place by clinicians working within the NHS, and particularly at the Tavistock Clinic in London, which supervises the treatment of all trans teenagers in the UK (excluding Northern Ireland) under the NHS.

These will include, as standard, a comprehensive clinical interview focused on gender identity, as well as extensive discussions between child, parents and psychologist. If anything, studies from the Netherlands suggest that because the criteria for prescribing puberty blockers to trans children are so strict it is more likely that individuals who would benefit from them do not receive them than vice-versa.

In addition, clinical protocols require that blockers should not be given until these young people have reached Tanner stage 2 or 3 of their original puberty. This is an objective standard, marked in male children by an enlargement of scrotum and testes, and a reddening/change in texture of scrotum skin. In female children, stage 2 includes breast budding, accompanied by some elevation of breast and papilla and enlargement of the areola.

The reason for waiting is that individual response to such changes is a good indicator of gender dysphoria, as well as a signpost to what treatment is appropriate. If the symptoms reduce with puberty, then it is likely that they are not suffering from gender dysphoria. If they persist and/or become more marked, then this reinforces the diagnosis of dysphoria.

Critics of transgender medicine argue that there are risks implicit in the application of puberty blockers. There are two core arguments. First, some critics have argued that puberty blockers should not be viewed as reversible, because all young people who take blockers will inevitably go on to transition. A more subtle form of this argument is that early administration of puberty blockers may have some effect on the natural development of a child's gender identity. This then makes it more likely that they will transition when without this early intervention they would not have.

The short answer – to both of these claims – is that they are patently false and that critics are demonstrating no more than their ability to ask a question. 'Do young people placed on puberty blockers *always* go on to transition?' The answer from several respected peer-reviewed studies is a straightforward no. A small but regularly reported cohort of teens placed on puberty blockers withdraw each year.

But could it still be the case that puberty-blocking treatment makes it more probable for these youth to retain their transgender identity, when experiencing their original puberty may have led some of them to adopt a cisgender identity? This too is unlikely.

Again, what evidence exists suggests quite the contrary. Research amongst teams working with trans youth drew a blank in respect of this concern. A direct study of brain function also found no evidence for this: quite the opposite, in that if any effect was present it appeared to be that puberty suppression tended to push brain functioning closer to natal sex. In other words, it made transitioning ever so slightly *less* likely!

Endocrinologists have also looked at outcomes following 'precocious puberty'. This is a medical condition in which puberty may start for a child at a distressingly early age, and for which puberty blockers have been used for many years. They reported being aware of absolutely no cases of gender dysphoria resulting from the administration of puberty blockers.

What about direct side-effects? As with any medical intervention, it is impossible to rule out entirely the possibility of side-effects and unintended consequences. There are some concerns that puberty blockers may slightly affect bone density and height. However, as the latter is an effect that many of those using puberty blockers are hoping for, that may be classified in many cases as a positive side-effect.

Absent from the public debate on whether to use puberty blockers is much – or even any – consideration of the downside of *not* using them. The question asked, repeatedly, by media pundits and TV people is: What if someone regrets it? Outwardly a fair question – until one remarks that statistics for trans regret are significantly lower than for other procedures, including abortion and prostate cancer treatment.

However, the question not asked is: What if they do not change their mind? If the result of intervention on the side of caution is to postpone or prevent treatment at puberty, then the trans individual is condemned either to a succession of seriously painful surgeries, or a life on the edge, never quite passing.

For trans men, the issues are different but no less serious. Adult height is determined in large degree by height at the onset of puberty. One way to view this is to see puberty as launch pad. The further you climb up a diving board, the more height you will achieve when you finally launch. Those who dive off earlier – who climb only to the first or second level before launching – will never go as high as those who climb to the very top before launching themselves off.

This is the issue that puberty blockers were first applied to. This was nothing to do with trans individuals, but dwarfism. Some variants of this condition originate with children launching into puberty at an early age, sometimes as young as four or five. Because puberty starts from such a low base in terms of physical development, individuals with this condition will never achieve the adult height they might otherwise have done. Puberty blockers help and in some cases avert this outcome completely.

Cis men tend to launch into puberty later than cis women, allowing for additional growth in terms of bodily bulk and height before puberty fixes them into their adult form. While shorter men are obviously not less masculine, trans men who undergo a full female puberty before transitioning will end up shorter, as men, than they would have had they made use of puberty blockers.

Separately, puberty brings on many other bodily changes, including breast growth and associated systems: changes to the areola, redistribution – or addition – of body fat. At transition, mastectomy is a well-tried procedure for which much experience exists. But if someone is unlikely ever to want breasts, then forcing them to go ahead and grow them – to undergo what for them may be an incredibly humiliating experience, only then, later, to remove them – is cruel.

In general, a wealth of literature suggests strongly that trans teens who are able to access puberty blockers have improved mental health outcomes and better quality of life. Those who do not receive such treatment are at quantifiably greater risk of depression, self-harm and suicidal behaviour. In addition:

- Individuals with untreated/unrecognised dysphoria have a tendency towards negative outcomes significantly above average for the general population. Untreated dysphoria is reported as associated not only with increased suicide risk, but also with a range of other psychosocial ailments, including alcoholism/drug abuse, depression and reduced ability to fit in to society.
- Where treatment is delayed, this risk persists post-treatment, with a strong correlation between the lateness at which treatment was begun and outcome.

In other words – and mirroring effects noted with other wholly unrelated treatments – the sooner that an individual feels that they are being taken seriously, and the sooner intervention is taking place to support them on their transition journey, the more likely they are to have a positive outcome. In fact, those treated early, and able to undergo a puberty close to the puberty they would have had in their identified gender, turn out as better adjusted and far more like non-trans children.

Diane Ehrensaft, a San Francisco psychologist specialising in the treatment of trans kids spoke about this in a recent interview. Talking of her direct experiences with one trans child, Nikki, she said:

> The kids that I work with, who know that they're going through puberty, that they're transgender, and therefore many of them are already socially transitioned, they're

looking like they're having a good time they hit this age 12–13 when everybody's bodies are changing and you start to think about your future a bit and they don't tank but they slope down and I just saw it in Nikki.

When you get to this age you start being able to think abstractly, you can think in larger constructs, you have a different sense therefore of yourself…you have to deal with reality, you just don't know what reality means, in this case we have a girl who doesn't have a uterus and wants to be a mommy, we have a girl who will grow breasts, but she hasn't gotten them yet and she has to do them by coming here to the clinic, and the reality of that has set in.

And then you start thinking about the romantic side, who's going to want me? In this case, I'm a girl with a penis, how am I going to do that? And so all of that I saw, right there in Nikki's kind of almost tearfulness, I'm not surprised I was a little sad myself to see Nikki in that slope down and I do think that what […] said was right, it will get better, and I think she knows that.

In respect of Synestra, her story highlights much that is wrong with the current level of education in the UK about LGBT issues. What now seems clear is that at an early age she was encouraged towards a self-identification as 'gay', as opposed to trans. She therefore received no treatment for her transness at an early age and underwent a full natal male puberty.

This, in turn, led her – logically – down a route of major, expensive and painful surgeries to rectify what puberty had wrought on her body. Just as logically, she made choices and lifestyle choices to pay for this work that were inherently risky. It is all too easy to play out 'what-if' scenarios. Syn's case highlights the benefits of more education and early awareness of trans identity.

Post-puberty

Following puberty, there are broadly two approaches to treating trans people who wish to align their body more closely to their understanding of it. The first is the use of cross-sex hormones to:

- block the uptake of those hormones that an individual's body is producing naturally; and
- encourage the development of secondary gender characteristics that align more closely with the gender identified.

For trans women, this involves some form of anti-androgen to block the production or uptake of testosterone, together with oestrogen to encourage the development of female features. For trans men, the hormone cocktail is reversed, with administration of testosterone.

Within the NHS, the use of cross-sex hormones is officially restricted to individuals aged 16 and over. However, existing protocols make it highly unlikely that an individual would be able to start such treatment the moment they reach 16. Other countries, most notably the US and Netherlands, have experimented with administering hormones earlier, on an informed consent or individual competency basis not dissimilar to that embodied in the principles of Gillick competence. The results appear to be significant positive outcomes for those so treated.

There is some evidence, mostly anecdotal, that one reason that clinics in the UK are unwilling to allow prescribing of hormones from an earlier age is directly linked to ideological campaigns designed to restrict access by young people to potentially life-saving treatments.

In addition, one Welsh GP, Dr Helen Webberley, has attempted to administer hormones on this basis at an earlier age. However, (see Chapter 4), this has brought her into conflict with the General Medical Council, and at time of writing she is subject to a disciplinary inquiry.

The NHS will pay for one part of the transition for trans women. Typically, that means hormones, from which it likely makes a small profit over the lifetime of the individual, plus testosterone blockers, which are slightly more costly.

The second approach post-puberty is surgery, as outlined above, to rectify some aspects of development brought about by puberty.

The NHS will fund genital surgery, the process historically referred to as 'gender re-assignment'. This includes some laser treatment, mostly to remove genital hair and to prevent an outcome in which the post-transition individual has in-growing hair in her newly constructed vagina, some voice therapy and some counselling. In practice, the last two are subject to a postcode lottery. Counselling is usually minimal, and not all areas offer voice therapy. In addition, a cricoid shave (a surgical process to reduce the Adam's apple) is usually available on the NHS.

Contrary to popular myth, a boob job is almost never available. It is viewed as a cosmetic procedure, and the NHS will not fund purely cosmetic treatments. A very few – a handful of trans women – have successfully pushed for such operations, and have been granted them on the same basis as a non-trans women. That is, where breast growth is negligible to non-existent and an independent psychologist report suggests that significant distress will be caused if such a procedure is not carried out. For those still tempted to assume that this means that all that is needed is a tame psychologist: the number of boob jobs carried out on trans women by the NHS over the last ten years is, at best guess, less than ten – perhaps less even than five.

It mostly does not happen. The total outlay on supporting a trans woman through hormones and surgery was estimated in 2012/13 at around £13,500; the outlay for trans men, who may undergo a wider range of more complex procedures, including mastectomy, etc. was estimated at the same time as closer to £60,000. However, not all trans men wish to undergo all of the procedures available.

In essence, this reflects the fact that cis interpretation of trans wants focuses almost wholly on the genital area. It is a thoroughly misleading trope, contributing to popular misunderstanding that being trans is something to do with sexuality. Whereas as Syn's own vlogging makes clear, the truth is very different.

Syn's master plan

As we have seen, from 2012, Syn started to post with increasing clarity that she saw herself now as trans and that her previous identification as gay was a mistake. In January 2013, she opened up to her online followers about what she was doing and the logic behind it. On YouTube she provided a no-holds-barred discussion of the surgery that trans people seek and, more importantly, that Syn wanted.

These were, in order, facial feminisation surgery (FFS), breasts and sexual re-assignment surgery; or, as she put it, she wanted facial feminisation in order to look female *before* she tackled 'breasts and pussy'.

Why, fans asked her, take the risk and undergo the major trauma involved in FFS? She discussed her motivations for these procedures and the logic behind them in some depth across a number of YouTube broadcasts.

One motivator was simply that she wanted to look more beautiful. More than beautiful, though: Syn was not simply trying to look less manly or less 'ugly'; she was striving for perfection. Over all, though, was her fear that she didn't look like a woman.

Humans are completely programmed to recognise male/

female, and Syn wanted to pass. If she just asked someone on the street whether she passed, it would be very difficult, because there are dozens of things that set out gender, from voice to moves, to behaviour. When we look at individuals we add up all of these factors, and come up with a result. A major influencer of that decision is how puberty creates a very clear differentiation between male and female faces because it changes skull shape.

Subtle differences include the brow ridging. Cues for maleness include the fact that the bottom two thirds of face is longer, with the result that you end up with a longer nose/lip distance and bottom half. She explained how she had been using make-up to disguise this: the 'drippy gothic thing' under her eyes as well as overdrawing of the top lip line. Both make eye to lips distance look shorter. There was much that could be done with make-up to feminise an individual's face, but surgery corrects them physically.

Without make-up – or hair – in most cases the face, the skull shape of a natal male will tend to prompt identification as a male. The face and skull shape of a natal female will lead an observer to conclude that they are female.

As befits someone who had spent so much of her life focused on using make-up in order to look the way she wanted to, there is much in these broadcasts on how male and female faces differ and how we can tell the difference between male and female immediately, instinctively.

In the long term, Syn wanted to eliminate any obviously masculine features that would set her apart as trans or male. She did not believe she passed well, or even at all, as a girl, and this was very important to her. She was aware that facial features were a significant factor in how people reached a conclusion as to gender.

At the most extreme, she imagined how she would look if she

had leukaemia and lost all her hair. Even then, she would want still to be read as a woman. In a vlog in early 2013 she said: 'I want to be able to live as a woman and pass as a woman 100% of the time and facial feminisation will help that.' She added: 'So long as my face looks correct, then I will be happy.'

FFS was therefore her priority in terms of building up funds, but as the most expensive of the procedures she wanted, it was also the most difficult.

She was clear that she would get her chin height reduced, as well as have a lip lift. In addition, she was planning to get eyebrows lifted, and hairline lowered, in order to do away with the M-hairline that is typically male. She would also get her Adam's apple shaved and her skull shortened, so that she would end up with a more flowing, more female forehead.

What is interesting is how much thought went into this aspect of the feminisation process, how little into the rest. How much, even, other procedures were tacked on almost as embarrassing afterthoughts, as though, for all that her everyday life was based in the erotic, she still found it embarrassing to talk intimate detail.

So, she was not sure about 'how big to have my tits'. Most men, she noted, encouraged her towards C or B, with a few advocating for D or E. The women she spoke with, by contrast, suggested she go for D or DD. Ever pragmatic, she felt she was unlikely to have the skin to accommodate E, but she might opt for D, since she had broad shoulders, and a D cup would provide her with cleavage.

As for her pussy the only debate, as far as Syn was concerned, was whether to go for the NHS, which meant getting it free, or going private, which would mean more of a chance for a 'designer vagina'.

And that was that. About three quarters of a broadcast focused on reshaping her face. Another 20% took in her breasts. Genital surgery – the focus for much of the cis medical establishment – was mentioned almost as afterthought. A throwaway. She concluded: 'Is the NHS vagina going to be good enough?'

Because paying meant it might cost around £20,000. Yet she seemed to have next to no sense of what might, or might not, constitute 'good enough'. Perhaps this reflects how little value she assigned to the sex act itself.

Elsewhere she reveals that she has researched a little more, explaining to one questioner that if sex-reassignment surgery is done correctly and well, then the M2F transsexual is usually sensate and often able to achieve orgasm. But, she adds: 'I don't personally really care about orgasms anyway... I find the topic somewhat boring. Sex for me is more about a mental gratification and pleasure, as opposed to a physical one.'

All this fits well with what Dani remembers of her. Dani reckons that 'if Syn were alive today, she would still be on the surgeon's table'. She understood transition in a way that was different from any trans woman Dani had ever known. She would study stuff down to its core, being as able to quote da Vinci's scientific schemes of gender when it came to assessing masculine and feminine features, as dealing with the technicalities of modern surgical techniques.

With her face, she would tinker and tinker and tinker. Her gender operation, which she never referred to as gender re-assignment was always going to be her last surgery.

For the rest, Syn was, for the time, perfectly satisfied. Unlike many trans women, she quite enjoyed having broad shoulders. Although, as she points out, she was probably less broad than many thought because her waist was just 24″, which made the rest of her look broader by contrast. Her arms were no wider than most females'. Besides, her overall proportions, including narrow hips and a broad chest, were very desirable from a high fashion perspective. Also, broad shoulders, on their own, would not create any issues when it came to passing in the same way that her facial features might.

As for her hips, she was more than satisfied with what she had. She observed, perhaps facetiously, that if she were to consider any further work, it would be to have a rib removed rather than any adjustment to her hips. She added: 'If Barbie were a real woman her hips would be 28″ and her waist, 17″ [whereas] my hips are 35 right now... That measurement will increase with hormones while my waist is just getting smaller and smaller (24″ at the moment). I think 37 hips with a 21 inch waist would be wicked measurements for me.'

Yet even this fairly level-headed calculation of the pros and cons of what she wanted to achieve was not without its critics.

Why did she care whether others thought she was female or not? Asked one. Surely all that matters was whether Syn felt comfortable in her body: she 'should reevaluate [her] goals'.

Another expressed admiration for her make-up videos but, they objected, Syn was too preoccupied with looks: she seemed very shallow, talking about herself 'as if you are a boy just trying to look like a girl instead of a woman born in the wrong body. It's a shame, I really did like you & your videos before this.'

Others picked up on her overall look: didn't her 'gothicness' prevent her from being perceived that much more as a 'natural' woman?

Syn's response? Not at all; in fact, hinting again at an evolution in her style, most of her gothness was now reserved for club nights. Outside of that, she was conscious that sometimes her personal style and the fact that she looked androgynous was an obstacle to people 'getting' her gender. But even though her objective was to pass as female, she was not planning to sacrifice her style in the vague hope that normality might make her pass better.

Besides, while she had her doubts about the value of normality when it came to passing, she *knew* any attempt to fit in, to follow a more 'normal' pathway would make her less desirable in general, because 'literally every man I speak to thinks the gothic influenced girl is dead hot'.

Still, the nay-sayers were out in force, and it is not hard to detect a hint of exasperation. At times, she appeared to be arguing with her fans about why she didn't want to argue. In her vlog she makes clear that she is aware of the risks and still wishes to go forward and transition, no matter what people tell her. At one point, she seems to be using her audience as a sounding board. Because if she can justify her plans to those who don't think she should go ahead, that will help her understand better for herself why she is doing what she is doing.

Some of the memes that surface are familiar. For instance, the same old scepticism over genital surgery. One wrote: 'Are u aware of the fact that getting bottom surgery is gonna decrease ur client rate like...alot?'

Syn had little patience for this:

I'm really bored of people telling me not to get a pussy... It's something that's really important to me and it's just stupid receiving an inbox full of messages saying 'OMG PLEASE NOOO!!' about such a serious, personal and well-considered decision.

I don't care if me becoming a woman is going to make me less fetish and less attractive to trannylovers. For all the people it makes me less attractive to, I'll rest assured at least the same number of people will find me more attractive with a pussy. Frankly, at the moment, I'm escorting to pay for my transition. I probably wont do much work when I'm finished transitioning.

I'm trans because I was born male and would like to be
a female, not because I want to be a tranny.

There were also some, possibly from a radical feminist perspective,
who took issue with her language:

Odd how you use 'pussy' to describe a vagina, but you say
'penis' for your male member and not 'dick' or 'cock'. Like a
'pussy' is just a thing and not something that will be a part
of you for the remainder of your life.

Am I the only one who thinks no transexual should get
the full surgery until they're mature enough to say 'vagina'
instead of 'pussy' or 'cunt' or whatever slang? Terminology
is all personal but...seriously? Can't say 'vagina' then no.
You don't deserve one.

Another posed the same question, albeit more mildly: 'You are
aware that most women don't call it a pussy. You sound like a man
when you say that, even though your not.'

For connoisseurs of social convention, there is an interesting
sociology to this discussion. The precise use of words to describe
one's genitals will vary according to age, class and politics. For
starters, many women 'of a certain age' – indeed many similarly
aged men – would hesitate to refer to a woman's vagina using some
of the stronger slang terms available. Many younger women, by
contrast, have fully reclaimed it, and will tend to use 'cunt' most
times in preference to the v-word.

And yes, 'pussy' is viewed by many as infantilising. A nursery
word. Men split in terms of their word preference, with many
opting for the c-word because they are simply not aware that it
might give offence. Sometimes, they are aware and wish to shock.
For the inverse reason, a segment of the male population casts

around for an alternative – any alternative – that does not invoke either c- or v-words.

Trans women often betray earlier socialisation with a similar embarrassment. Yet many change the way they refer to themselves post-transition. When they have a vagina of their own, they are, as other women, far more matter of fact about it, and much more likely to use whatever word is in common currency amongst their own female friends.

Even so, there is no absolute rule. One of the most radical feminists I know is regularly given to alternating 'pussy' with 'cunt': she tends to reject the v-word as itself patriarchal in origin.

In other words, there is no clear answer: and trying to skewer a trans woman with a presumed social convention will not work.

Syn answered this in her own inimitable way: 'Only men say pussy? That is such nonsense.'

She went on: 'Maybe what you say is true amongst your friends, but in my life I do not believe it to be true at all and my life and geographical location is of no less importance or statistical value than yours. Personally, I think pussy is probably my favourite word for vagina.'

That said, this is no feminist perspective on Syn's behalf, but something deeply conventional for she concludes: '...different words for vagina exist and although they mean the same thing, they put a different spin on the sentence in which they are used. For example, if I wanted to convey filthy imagery I might choose the word "cunt" instead. If I were referring to the female genitals in academic writing I would use "vagina".'

Not everyone was a critic, and in the end, Syn may have drawn some strength from this commenter:

I say go for it. Your nose turned out amazing, so if your FFS goes just as well, you're going to be drop dead gorgeous.

Lets be honest, these bitches just don't want your hot ass as competition! It's your life, and you shouldn't listen to all to anyone that judges your choices on tumblr – like, omg there's nothing wrong with what you do and you shouldn't be shamed for it by prudish children.

Oh, & btw; I get it, the fact that you want to look like a woman without make-up too. I'm a woman, & very often I don't wear make-up, & I obviously still look like a woman. I've got short hair in a bob, & even when I've got it brushed back so it looks like a boyish cut (f.ex; if I'm crafting or something) & no make-up I still look like a woman. I think I would find it very upsetting if I _had_ to wear make-up & do my hair every day just for people to know that I'm a woman. So, I get that. :)

Endorsement indeed!

The price of desperation

If the NHS won't pay for it, then what is a trans woman to do?

Some sense of the lengths to which an individual will go – the sheer desperation – emerge from a story in September 2017. Unable to afford gender reassignment surgery, trans woman Lila Rose, originally from France, but now living in the UK, was offering her post-transition 'virginity' to the highest bidder.

The story was sensationalised in the *Sun* newspaper with suggestions that Lila was offering a 'mind blowing' sexual experience. However, interviewed by Gay Star News, Lila spoke of her anger at the way the *Sun* had reported her offer. They sensationalised and made her look cheap. Yet in the end, it was not even about the money, she says; rather, she 'just wanted to show people [her] struggle': 'It was an SOS for me and other girls like me who don't have enough money, we face discrimination all around the world. I am lucky that I live in Europe, but the waiting lists are still crazy. When you are in transition you just want it to be finished. 25 years of waiting, I just want to live my life. It's killing me, it's ruining my life.'

And that, in a nutshell, is the dilemma for many trans people. The NHS does offer support for some parts of the transition process – but only part – and the waiting times in some UK regions are excruciating. One region, in 2016, reported that waiting times for gender re-assignment surgery could lengthen, over the next few years, to 12 years. That is a long time if you are even mildly uncomfortable in your own body. It is next to impossible if your bodily dysphoria is more significant.

In 2015, the first major national Trans Beauty Pageant took place in the UK, to an accompaniment of criticism from the wider trans community. There were concerns that this reinforced stereotyped views of women and trans women. For the pageant included a talent section, in which judges voted on contestants according to their skill in a particular thing. However, the sense remained that such an event retained all the bad features of a more common cis beauty contest, with a (prurient) focus on the physical attributes of those taking part.

Well, yes. I attended, and I wrote about the event for the national press. Despite the best efforts of organisers, this was far from the most politically correct event of the year. Yet at the same time, I refused to join in the wider criticism.

There is a joke, within trans circles, about suitable occupations for trans women: either computer programming or sex work. The first, because it enables individuals to earn the money they need for transition without having to dare the workplace environment. It is an ideal solution for the educated, middle-class professional able to pivot the last vestiges of male privilege into speeding their journey onward. And the second is for those who lack the skills, the qualifications. Common to both is the possibility of making enough money to survive and transition without having to face the near inevitable disapproval of a hostile work environment.

Such explanations clearly would not wash for one anonymous critic who wrote: 'Noo...why do you spread your cheeks for money? Once I found you extremely enchanting and smart. I'm sorry, but the idea that everybody can buy you for some coins destroys all of your magic. Quick money = transgender sickness?'

Syn's answer to this, as to everything else was calm, cool, logical:

My priorities lie with becoming a woman. I desire to be passable, functional and, for all intents and purposes from the perspective of society, a female. This means I need to save money for surgical procedures... Prostitution and escorting is the quickest route to this monetary goal.

I do not believe in attributing intangible 'value' to the act of sex. In my mind, from an incredibly logical perspective, I see sex as basically a specific and defined co-ordination between two bodies. As far as I'm concerned with escorting, this means a homo sapiens organism embedding his genitalia within me.

This...costs me nothing but time... I am paid for this time, and subsequently, I become closer to my monetary goal and that means I will able to transition into the female which I so desire to become, sooner.

Do not feel sad that my body is used in exchange for money. My body is my body and until I am fully finished transitioning, my body will be currency for its own development. I actually gain satisfaction from the knowledge that the body I have now is actually going to be my route to the new body I wish to have.

The important thing to remember is that I am not a

victim of any kind. I choose this route and I do not begrudge it. I am happy to sell sex for money. If I found prostitution morally jarring with my beliefs (as some would) I would seek an alternate route to earning the money I need to earn. I am thankful that I am not incarcerated by moral inhibitions – I am thankful that I see the world in which I live in at face value. I do not try and give intimate acts like sexual intercourse more meaning than they deserve.

This is her manifesto: heartfelt and personal. Yet, reading it, one cannot help but hear echoes of every trans person who has ever struggled, without support, without independent means, to achieve their lifelong goal of transition.

Syn's uniqueness was that she had the beauty, the charisma and the single-mindedness to make it work.

CHAPTER 4

Seeking Help

So much for the master plan. It all sounds so logical as Syn sets it out. Yet the practice, at least in relation to her interaction with the NHS, was never going to be easy and, as matters turned out, this was going to be her downfall.

Let's start with the surgeries. It does not take long, watching and listening to Syn, to realise how important it was to her to be admired and desired: almost everything was done in order to be the centre of attention. As one close friend observed, she always dressed well, but that was illusion. She did not buy expensive clothes, ever, because she was desperate to transition. So she saved every bit of money she could for that single goal.

That is not a uniquely trans thing: think, rather, aspiring movie star, Marilyn Monroe. It is a way of being and of looking at life that afflicts some (young) people, trans and otherwise. A few – a very few – eventually make their way through the auditions and past the casting couch to achieve fame and celebrity in their own right. The vast majority fall by the wayside. Syn, from her early teens, had achieved some minor celebrity and as she grew older, it was clearly her intention to draw down the dividends from that.

As revealed in Chapter 3, her priorities were all about her look, rather than her genitals, and so it was surgically. The following dates are as accurate as possible, but as they are compiled from the recollections of other people, they may not be entirely accurate:

- She started with a nose job in June 2012.
- Next stop was a lip lift in August 2013.
- A boob job followed in January 2014.
- Finally, Syn underwent full facial feminisation, including a forehead 'peel', brow lift and tracheal shave in August 2014.

The difference was startling: a mix of subtle and less subtle. The boob job almost certainly fell in the latter category. Those who know her, as well as anyone who is interested enough in Syn's story to seek out pictures of her online, must judge for themselves. However, between 2012 and 2015 it is possible to watch a gradual transition from a look designed for the clubs and with much in common with fetish and drag performance, to a softer, more feminine look.

In addition, according to Lux, Syn was undergoing electrolysis – most decidedly *not* a cheap procedure – and had had dermal fillers applied. Also, while Syn appears not to have mentioned this to anyone, her voice, in her later broadcasts had softened and feminised. That is something that an individual can achieve through their own efforts – but with great difficulty. More likely, Syn had had some help from a specialist in this field.

All told, Lux estimates that Syn spent somewhere between £30k and £50k on transition procedures – and likely at least in the middle of this range. Unclear is whether this was on top of hormone spend which, by Syn's own estimates would have added several thousand more from 2012 onward. Going it alone as a trans woman with high standards is not cheap!

There were also considerable risks to this approach that surprisingly – given her extensive research in other areas – Syn had not obviously taken into account. Already noted are concerns over self-prescribing anti-androgens and hormones from the internet. Not only is one never quite sure of the potency or the authenticity of the substance one is taking, but one is not, unless paying for independent monitoring, undergoing basic checks. These serve a dual purpose, ensuring that the desired hormone levels are being reached, and also that there are no side-effects or contra-indications. These are of low likelihood, but nonetheless complications can arise in terms of liver function and possible cardiac episodes.

A further complication is the dangers of a 'too-early' boob job. That is, in fitting breast implants in the first two to three years on feminising hormones, while these are still actively producing growth. The issue is self-evident: if you insert a relatively massive implant at a point in time when the final shape of an individual's breasts is not yet settled, then it is impossible to say what the final result will be. The growing breast tissue may form around the implant: or there may be some conflict between the two, leading to an unsightly result. In the worst-case outcome, a too-early implant can cause nerve and circulation problems and even damage the breast, requiring removal of the implant.

If Synestra commenced taking hormones, as she suggests, in early 2012, and continued the course without interruption and, additionally, if these hormones were of the appropriate strength and dosage to her transition, then no harm done. But if any of these conditions was not met, there could have been problems with her breasts later on.

As it was, she managed successfully to negotiate the majority of possible surgical procedures on her own and with little or no assistance from the NHS. The end results were superficially pleasing, and there were no obvious side-effects.

Still, from the outset, Syn wanted her treatment brought inside the NHS. It is not entirely clear why. It would not have saved her any money – at least not in respect of the surgical treatments she had. Almost none of her surgeries, with the possible exception of the tracheal shave, are available on the NHS as they are regarded as primarily for cosmetic purposes. She was always going to have to pay for facial feminisation.

Those close to her have suggested a number of possible reasons. Inside the NHS she would have been able to obtain her hormones on prescription, and this would eventually have constituted a significant saving to her, but minor cost to the NHS, over the years. It would also guarantee the quality of the hormones she was taking.

She would also, eventually, have been eligible for gender re-assignment surgery (GRS). Whether she would have wanted an 'NHS job' is another issue entirely. What the NHS provides 'down there' is adequate both urologically and neurologically. That is, NHS surgeons will remove existing genital structures (including penis and testes), reconnect the 'plumbing' (to ensure that post-op the individual is able to pee without difficulty), and reconnect nerves to the small amount of penile tissue used to constitute a clitoris, so as to give the post-op trans woman a reasonable chance of still being able to achieve orgasm.

What the NHS does not do is a cosmetic job. Post-op, the 'finish' to the newly minted trans vulva will vary greatly. It is unlikely, however, to approximate the 'porn star vagina' look that is the trademark of surgeons whose training has been in plastic surgery. And it is the latter that one will tend to get if one goes private.

A pre-op visit to one's NHS surgeon in the UK will cover basics, and risks, and recovery period and procedures that the trans woman will need to undergo. The equivalent visit to a private clinic in, say Thailand, where a significant number of gender re-assignment procedures are carried out, is more likely to end with the patient flicking through a vagina catalogue and discussing with the surgeon how they would like to look after the event.

For many, it is a surreal moment, being asked to map out the contours of their future genitals. It is certainly not for everyone. Some do not care. Some are icked or embarrassed by the very idea, happy to submit to the English surgical knife so long as the end result is passable – and almost always it is. There is immense variety in how cis women look.

Yet there is cultural pressure towards the idealised 'porn star' look: far more similarity than natural variation on display in the pages of the average porn magazine. And trans women are no different to their cis sisters. Those who can afford to pay for 'beauty', 'normality', or whatever other label they place on a look, often do so. Those who cannot take what they can get.

As one trans businesswoman wrote, you only do this (transition) once in your lifetime. So if you are going to do this, you need to do it right. She, like Syn, had money to spend, and estimated her final budget on transition at well in excess of £50,000 – a decade or so before Syn started to transition.

Syn's own estimate of the surgical cost would have taken her personal transition up past the £70,000 mark – though it is possible she erred on the high side. Broadly speaking, there is cost equivalence between GRS in the UK and in a Far Eastern country such as Thailand. In the UK, the cost of gender re-assignment, including an anaesthetist and relatively luxurious private clinic will set you back about £11,000.

A few years back, it was estimated that taking into account the cost of flights and private nursing, the cost of GRS in Thailand was about the same. The surgery component was likely to cost no more than about £6500, with flights, after-care and accommodation taking up the balance.

Syn's estimate, of £20,000, suggests either she hadn't budgeted quite as precisely for her GRS as she had for other procedures or she was considering additional work. Although it is hard to imagine what more she could have had done.

So coming into the NHS would have saved her £10,000; possibly, in her own mind, as much as £20,000.

But she was looking to come back on board as early as 2012 – was visiting gender specialists and attempting to obtain a referral to a gender identity clinic from the earliest days of her transition. This suggests that in addition to the cost element, she felt the NHS could provide something she could not provide for herself. Guidance, perhaps. A useful backstop, in case of complications, as well as a legitimacy that she could not obtain on her own.

Perhaps she just wanted someone else in charge: someone to take responsibility. However, getting into the system was, in the end, to prove one of the few challenges that got the better of her.

NHS ecosystem

In Chapter 3, we highlighted the stages that an individual seeking a full binary transition is likely to undergo. Ideally, they would understand, from early puberty, that the possibility of transition existed and receive treatment, including counselling, support and – medically – puberty blockers.

From age 16, the individual will be permitted, if it is considered appropriate, to take cross-gender hormones. From 18, surgery becomes an option. These are, broadly, the ages at which such procedures are available on the NHS and also, increasingly, the ages at which they can be accessed privately, both in the UK and internationally.

The majority of countries where gender re-assignment surgery (increasingly referred to as gender confirmation surgery) is now carried out will require that the individual be 18 or over, in line with World Professional Association for Transgender Health (WPATH) guidelines on the treatment of gender dysphoria. The exception is mastectomy (the removal of breast tissue), which may be carried out in respect of trans men from age 16 onward.

There is less agreement on the appropriate age at which to administer cross-sex hormones. In the UK, the NHS has mostly held fast to 16 as the age at which this is permissible, with one or two practitioners pushing for GPs to have the right to prescribe hormones earlier if they feel it is in the best interests of the patient.

If the processes and stages that a trans person is likely to undergo medically are relatively well known and well set-out, there are nonetheless hurdles that they must overcome in order to receive treatment – at least within the NHS. These are subject to a bitter medico-political argument between centralising tendencies (gender specialists), and an increasingly unwilling sharp-end service (GPs). Meanwhile, private services, which have historically been able to fill gaps, are at increasing risk from a power grab by the centre.

At the time when Synestra first sought help, the route was rather longer and more complex than now. An individual looking for NHS support would need to persuade their GP of this, and they, in turn would make a referral either directly to a gender identity clinic (GIC), of which there are a dozen in the UK (at time of writing: seven in England, four in Scotland, one in Northern Ireland and none in Wales) or to a local mental health team, whose role was to pre-screen potential patients, eliminating those with major psychiatric disorder, before referring on to a GIC.

This process has now been considerably shortened with the possibility, since 2013 for GPs in England, to refer patients directly to a GIC without the need for a mental health assessment first (a stage that often added between six and 18 months to the process).

GICs will then assess the individual, deciding whether they consider them to be gender dysphoric or not, and set about dispensing treatment: hormones and, eventually, surgery. Depending on what funding is available, GICs may also pay for some laser treatment prior to surgery, and some voice training. The GIC will also manage referrals on to other specialist services within the NHS: for instance, to endocrinologists, to monitor hormone levels.

While this is all positive, the journey to the GIC remains long and arduous. Wait time to first appointment is at least 12 to 18 months, depending on what part of the country one lives in. And then treatment will not commence before a second interview. So the wait from referral to treatment is frequently two to three years. Thereafter, surgery may take place within one year of commencement of hormones (according to WPATH guidelines); though English GICs will not put anyone forward for recommendation at less than two years. Scottish ones may put them forward sooner.

In the North-East region, however, a stark warning was issued in 2015 that waiting time for surgery could eventually reach 12 years.

GICs also have an ambivalent reputation within the trans community. On the one hand, they have their fans. They are, after all, for anyone unable to afford the cost of treatment privately, the only real option and for many a life-saver. At the same time, they are seen as gate-keepers, introducing barriers to treatment in part to sustain their own position as dispensers of expertise.

Historically, too, the relationship has been problematic. One criticism often levelled at trans individuals – trans women especially – is that they reinforce both gender stereotypes and the gender binary. The unfairness of this accusation is felt deeply within the trans community, as in the early days, access to treatment was conditional on fitting clinician preconceptions about gender binary.

There were countless examples of individuals refused treatment because they were too tall, or married, because they wore insufficiently feminine clothes or their posture and mannerisms did not fit the accepted gender model.

Also problematic was insistence by GICs that transition

should be a binary process: a journey from male to female or vice-versa. Individuals who only wanted a partial transition (more common amongst trans men, for whom transition consists of multiple independent processes) would be rejected as 'not trans enough'. The recent growth in non-binary, both in terms of public awareness and assertiveness by those who identify as such, mean this has reduced.

While the bulk of (trans)gender-related services take place in the GICs, there is a significant debate going on currently around two issues. First, the extent to which gender services can be delivered via GPs, and how far they need to be delivered by specialist services. Second, the extent to which gender services can or should be provided privately and in non-standard ways.

At present, GPs interact with trans patients in a number of ways. As already noted, until recently, they had a role in referring the trans patient onward to the GIC. However, GPs may provide support for trans individuals in a number of additional ways. When they first arrive at their GP, seeking help for gender dysphoria, they may, as in Synestra's case, already be 'self-medding': that is, acquiring hormones through a variety of sources, some more legal than others, and medicating themselves.

According to the General Medical Council (GMC), GPs should be prepared to issue 'bridging prescriptions' in some exceptional circumstances – for example, if patients were already on self-medicated hormonal treatments – as a means to minimise the risk of self-harm or suicide. The thinking behind this is analogous to programmes designed to wean individuals off dangerous/unlawful drugs. They provide an alternative safe and tested source, within a framework that means that their use, as well as any side-effects, can be monitored.

Historically, too, it has been common practice for trans patients to receive an initial diagnosis from a private specialist, who may prescribe hormones, together with a reassurance that their GP will then take on their prescription and monitor their treatments.

This is not without pushback from some GPs. In a recent *Guardian* piece,[3] a GP argued that the GMC guidance was at best misleading. To begin with, the GMC recommended that GPs should seek specialist advice from a GIC. However, if this was not possible and a GP did not feel able to prescribe with confidence, then it suggested seeking advice from a GIC and/or the local clinical commissioning group.

Pushback came in the form of a number of points made by this author. It was difficult, they argued, to ascertain precisely what 'exceptional circumstances' are. Besides, gender dysphoria was a niche field. Patients needed specific management with 'a multi-disciplinary team approach that encompasses endocrinologists, surgeons, psychiatrists, pharmacists and others'. This, though, was beyond the capacity of GPs to provide due to the constraints already existing in offer in their 'time-poor and under-resourced primary care'.

The advice from NHS England is also that GPs should undertake this work, including monitoring treatments through blood and hormone levels. Contradicting this, the British Medical Association's General Practitioner Committee has warned GPs not to prescribe specialised treatments, as they might thereby fail to provide holistic care to gender dysphoria patients, with the result that GPs risk an increase in complaints.

In short, the issue of prescribing and specialised support was contentious and, this GP wrote: 'Gender dysphoria patients deserve better treatment than I can give them.'

They add: 'Deficiencies in the commissioning of gender

---

3   www.theguardian.com/society/2017/aug/15/gender-dysphoria-patients-need-specialists-not-gps

dysphoria services need to be tackled urgently. GPs who aren't gender identity specialists are not best placed to fill that role safely and effectively, yet we still carry the responsibility for our prescribing. However, any reticence on our part to prescribe can be challenged and can sometimes be misinterpreted for prejudice.'

The piece ends with an appeal to the NHS to sort out both the commissioning and support structures available to treat gender dysphoria. The author welcomes the public consultation that is being carried out through 2017 in terms of developing a gender support service for the future, and appears to look forward positively to a future in which GPs are supported by regional GICs and specialist GP groups. This is all very positive and, if the author truly means it, is admirable.

However, many in the trans community expressed concern that this was special pleading dressed up as 'in the best interests of the trans community'. In modern parlance, 'concern trolling'. There are several reasons for this suspicion.

To begin, the author of this piece writes dismissively of individuals turning up at their GPs with prescriptions from private specialists, and expecting GPs to take over such prescriptions. Perhaps they are right to be suspicious of such shortcuts – although the practice of taking over prescriptions from specialists in other areas is commonplace. Indeed, much specialist treatment would simply seize up if GPs were to take this approach across the board. In discipline after discipline, GPs accept that they are not specialists but that once a specialist has done their job and prescribed, there is some obligation on them to take over treatment.

Second, while the author is keen to re-assure that GPs have no objection to taking on prescriptions where these are underpinned by recognised (NHS) specialist groups, history suggests that is not the case. For GPs also feature within the trans universe after individuals have been accepted for treatment by a GIC and have been prescribed hormones by that GIC. The current structure of the NHS means that GICs do not have a drugs budget – so all they can do is prescribe. Historically, this has worked with GPs administering hormones under a 'shared care' agreement: the GIC writes a letter, and the GP does as asked.

In recent years, however, there has been increasing pushback from GPs in respect of not-approved drugs. They have a right not to prescribe anything they are not entirely happy with, and lack of official approval is as good a reason as any. A 'not-approved drug' in this context is any drug that has not been tested and specifically approved for a particular purpose.

Unfortunately, there are almost no drugs approved for transition purposes. This is because the trans community is relatively tiny and the drugs used – typically hormones – are low cost. A few pounds per prescription: in some cases, a few pence. Whereas the cost of implementing a specific testing programme can run into many millions of pounds.

So transgender drugs are not approved. They are simply drugs that have been tested for other purposes – for hormone replacement therapy, for instance, in women – and repurposed for transition. While this sounds alarming, and the spectre of 'untested drugs' has been used as yet another stick with which to beat the trans community, it is far more theoretical than real.

Formal testing is intended primarily to achieve two objectives: to establish the risk profile, including side-effects, of the drug being tested; and to show that it will produce the intended effect as well as or better than existing alternatives and at a comparable or lower cost.

Hormones: best practice in action

An individual, transitioning in middle age, decided to short-circuit the transition process by going to a private consultant. They agreed a diagnosis of gender dysphoria and after a period of real-life experience – WPATH guidelines require this and/or psychiatric evaluation before treatment is administered – issued a first prescription for hormones. This private prescription cost the patient £120, including a nominal amount for an additional consultation.

Thereafter, the prescription was taken over by the individual's GP. This was discussed in depth with the GP and, since she had some concerns over the acceptable limits of hormone prescribing, a referral was made to an endocrinologist within the NHS: in fact not just any endocrinologist, but an expert in the use of hormones in treating trans patients.

The endocrinologist was able to do two things. In the first instance, he evaluated the hormones being used and confirmed that the amount of hormone prescribed was reasonable and could continue without issue. In addition, he provided guidelines for hormone use and, more importantly, gave the GP additional information – a checklist – on what tests should be carried out on a regular basis, what to look for, and what could go wrong with hormone prescription (not a lot, but not 100% without possible drawbacks).

This proved especially useful when, after some years of settling nicely around the recommended target range, this patient's oestrogen levels decided to head off the chart. This was unlikely to prove fatal, but it was definitely the sort of thing that needed to be kept under review.

This was picked up at regular tests carried out by the GP: hormone dose adjusted – twice, in the end – and thereafter micro-managed, again, without need for expensive consultant sessions, and without any need for the individual to take a day off work travelling to London to spend 20 minutes, perhaps less, in the office of an expert.

In the case of hormones, the most common treatment for trans individuals, there is now a long history – decades of hormone prescription – with no major side-effects showing up. Oestrogen, which Synestra was taking, is prescribed regularly for millions of non-trans women every year with next to no questions asked.

In practice, when a woman reaches a certain age and is presumed to be menopausal or pre-menopausal, the average GP will simply ask whether they would like hormone replacement therapy (HRT), and if the answer is yes, a prescription will be issued. In some cases, this will be followed up with monitoring of hormone levels – but not always. There are known side-effects and, as with all other medication, patients are instructed to watch out for such and to return to the GP should such side-effects show up. They are not required to undergo extensive psychiatric evaluation beforehand!

In recent years, however, trans patients have had increasing problems with this arrangement. In some instances, GPs have exercised their right, as set out above, not to prescribe where they are not themselves 100% sure of the merits of the drug being prescribed. In others, there has been unseemly toing and froing over the budget, with both GPs and GICs claiming they have no funds to pay for treatment. Some trans patients have, as a result, found themselves in limbo for months, while GP and GIC play medical ping-pong. This is hardly a clever way to treat an individual who, as the author of the *Guardian* article cited above readily admits, can become depressed and suicidal if left untreated.

In some parts of the country, there are now very definite trans 'no-go' areas. Practices where all of the GPs have decided that they will not prescribe transition hormones and where trans patients must either complain officially if they want to receive any treatment or transfer to another practice. Yet even this will not do in some cases, for some of these are entire NHS areas. Some boroughs, some commissioning groups, have seen GPs agree between themselves that they will collectively refuse to prescribe cross-gender hormones.

All of this merely reinforces a sense within the trans community that while some GPs may have genuine concerns in this respect, the real reason why many will not prescribe is rather more straightforward: a personal ethical objection to the very principles of transgender treatment.

#TransDocFail

This sense that GPs do not have the best interests of trans patients at heart is further added to by a campaign, an issue, known as #TransDocFail. This was, in origin, a spontaneous outpouring of trans anger and disgust aimed at the medical profession as a result of what many considered to be a General Medical Council vendetta against one trans-friendly medic, Dr Richard Curtis.

But more of that later.

The spur to this anger was a sense, quite contrary to that alluded to by the article about GP dilemmas in treating trans patients, that the trans community as a whole was getting a raw deal from the UK medical establishment – and not just when it came to specifically trans issues, such as referrals to gender identity clinics or the prescribing of hormones.

Rather, they were being discriminated against pretty much across the entire spectrum of medical treatment.

So people began to tweet out their personal stories on Twitter. Then, as the seriousness of what was being revealed began to sink in, a number of campaigners formalised these complaints. They took fuller histories from those telling their story, collated them, forwarded them to the General Medical Council.

To give a better idea of why the trans community as a whole

does not greatly trust medical practitioners, below is just a selection of the stories told. These are taken from #TransDocFail tweets collated by Cambridge city councillor Zoe O'Connell on her site, and represent just a sub-set of that sub-set.

To begin with, there is the difficulty in obtaining treatment: one NHS GP refused to believe a trans patient when she informed them that she was seeing an endocrinologist on the NHS because 'all that trans stuff is only available privately'. Another told a trans individual asking about treatment that they had never heard of gender dysphoria and 'The NHS definitely doesn't do that'.

The same patient (post-transition) was later treated with hostility by their gynaecologist, was asked if they 'regretted it' and told that most trans women eventually detransition anyway. Many stories emerged of doctors and psychiatrists either refusing to refer patients for treatment, or making excuses for not doing so. Even in the last few years, the old cliché that an individual could not transition unless they would make a passable woman (or man) at the end of the process remained common.

Support – and funding – for various treatments was patchy. Most controversial was electrolysis, which many NHS trusts refused to fund because it was 'cosmetic'. That is arguable when electrolysis is sought in respect of an individual's face; not so when the electrolysis is to be applied to donor tissue prior to vaginoplasty.

In plain English, some skin – usually scrotal tissue – that was previously on the outside of the body will end up inside as result of vaginoplasty. Without electrolysis of that area, trans women who have gender re-assignment surgery may end up with internal 'hair balls'. These are prone to infection, uncomfortable and in at least two cases of which this author is aware, so seriously debilitating that the patient was unable to walk.

Nonetheless, this procedure was deemed cosmetic. So, too, was rectifying a botched breast augmentation job gone so badly wrong that the patient was left with constant, serious and incapacitating pain. Rather than treat the actual issue, the local hospital recommended the individual for 'pain management'.

All of this, of course, happened in addition to or around the struggle that many trans patients had simply to get their GP to put them forward to a gender identity clinic in the first place. While the *Guardian* article mentioned above expressing concern for trans patients refers to average waiting times of 12 to 18 months, this does not take into account delay that seems to arise for almost any reason and none.

Five years from seeing GP to getting surgery (that was a comparatively good outcome); three years waiting for a GIC appointment (during which time the individual started self-medding); 44 months from first seeing GP to GIC. Some of this, undoubtedly, has to do with demand for GIC services. Much, though, does not. Individuals told of referrals to psychotherapy going missing (one for over a year): referrals left on the GP's desk and not forwarded; the GP who repeatedly told a patient they had referred them to a GIC (they hadn't!).

The matter-of-fact GP who told a trans woman to 'pull yourself together and stop wasting my time'; the teenage client asked by their doctor to wait a year because then they would be at university and 'the doctor there can deal with it'; another told to 'focus on their disability', because that was what was really important.

Stories of GPs refusing to administer treatment (hormones) even where prescribed by a GIC are legion. One refused to prescribe HRT even after they had been recommended by a GIC because of concerns that the patient was 'not taking them safely' – not a consideration that regularly seems to enter into the doctor–patient dialogue.

Other refusals appear simply cruel, if not downright dangerous. For instance, a pre-op trans man who, after being on hormones for three years, had them stopped by their GP. Another trans woman tells of how her GP just withdrew post-op HRT without asking her. This comes close to serious malpractice. For whatever the rights and wrongs of placing a trans person on hormones, once on, and especially post-op, their withdrawal can have serious adverse consequences, both medical and psychological.

Not just GPs either. There was the individual refused hormones by their endocrinologist because they weren't wearing 'women's clothing': this, apparently, meant they weren't being serious.

Then there were GPs who were just obstructive. One GP refused to write a letter stating that a trans woman had had surgery (this was requested to enable her to obtain a gender recognition certificate). Another refused to write a letter to say they lived full-time as male because 'only an endocrinologist' could certify that (not true). Many simply refused treatment. One, it is alleged, refused treatment and then, likely in contravention of the law, shredded the patient's notes.

Despite the suggestion that gender issues are specialised and that GPs are not qualified to deal with them, there is the 'GP knows best' tendency. This often takes the form of 'You're really gay' or 'You're too young', or even 'It's your mother'. There was the young person who went to talk with their GP about gender dysphoria. Their GP told them there's 'nothing wrong with being gay', before sending them to a family planning clinic. Another told a trans woman she wasn't really trans because she played Dungeons & Dragons and this (their female persona) was just another new character.

There was the GP who reduced an individual's hormone dosage because they (the GP) decided that they needed greater libido. They didn't ask first! Another objected to a trans person who said they had no interest in genital surgery, arguing that 'sex is very important to some people'. This ignored the individual's clear and thought-out sense of their own sexuality, as well as imposing a highly cisnormative view of what sexuality entailed.

Many GPs simply refuse to recognise genders that fall outside their idea of what constitutes the norm, refusing to discuss or acknowledge non-binary models of gender. In more than one instance, being non-binary was cited as a reason for refusing HRT.

A further common complaint is the failure of NHS systems to be able to update records to accommodate new names, titles and genders properly. Or rather, the failure, mostly, of practice systems. One of the most frustrating issues for trans people is going through a lengthy process to change their details at one point in the NHS – only to have the wrong name or gender pop up unexpectedly somewhere else. Though this assumes that mistakes *are* administrative, and not some form of deliberate misgendering or 'outing'.

NHS policy is to change name, title and sex on patient record on demand. However NHS staff in one facility simply refused to believe this. In fact, it is relatively easy to change name within the overall NHS system. However, because GPs operate computer systems independent of central records, change is not always automatically carried through. Many practice systems are anyway far less adaptable. One trans person, for instance, reveals how they were told by their GP that it was not possible to change gender marker at surgery and title was gender-linked.

Individuals routinely tell of GPs who insist on using a former name even when their name has been updated on systems. Worst of all are instances – too many to list – where patients are outed, on forms, in doctor to doctor conversations, to nurses or even, to the entire community, as doctors or receptionists call patients in to appointments using their old name.

Perhaps, therefore, the *Guardian* writer and 'trans deserve better' apologist is unaware of the true horror stories. First off is the issue of the 'transsexual broken arm' – at other times known as the 'transexual cold'. When a trans patient arrives at their GP's surgery (or even in their A&E) it would appear that nothing can be done to treat even the most banal and non-trans of ailments – because they are trans!

One individual was denied treatment for a cardiac condition because with 'all this gender stuff going on so it was probably in my head'. Another reported a practitioner (in A&E) insisting on carrying out a genital exam before giving a chest X-ray for chest pain. Many trans people reported being turned down for mental health support for conditions wholly unrelated to their gender dysphoria: sometimes because they were being seen at a GIC, sometimes because mental health issues were assumed to be obvious consequence of the dysphoria.

Routine gynaecological and other issues are frequently escalated to local hospitals or back to the GIC 'because the patient is trans'. One patient reported almost every issue they have being assumed, by their GP, to be a side-effect of HRT. Another had serious physical symptoms dismissed as psychosomatic 'because they were trans'. Routine appointments about matters as distinct as hearing and bad back are regularly turned into discussions of gender and/or hormone treatment.

While that is bad, it gets worse. NHS fetishisation of trans people leads on either to abuse or to dangerously abusive treatment. One individual told of the time they were taken to a local hospital having lost two pints of blood after their gender re-assignment surgery. Nothing happened – other than that this became a prime opportunity for nurses to gather round and discuss transness.

There were multiple reports of simple degrading verbal abuse. One individual was turned away at the reception of their local gynaecological clinic and described as 'it' as they did so. A trans man was told he only wanted to transition to male because he was too ugly to live as a women. The wife of a trans woman was told by a sexual health clinic that she was at high risk for AIDS/STIs because she 'has sex with transgenders'. Another trans woman was referred to as a 'shemale' – for most trans people a highly insulting term – by their psychotherapist.

A great many unnecessary genital examinations. Not to mention the individual told it was a shame how so much effort was put into trans treatment while there was no cure for cancer. Or the individual who rang NHS Direct to obtain help for their partner. The NHS Direct doctor spoke to their partner and told them to leave the first caller, as they were an 'abomination'.

The patient with a perforated appendix refused a wheelchair by hospital staff: forced to walk to the operating theatre; later told that they could have died as a result of that single piece of discrimination.

Within the space of a few weeks, the hashtag attracted several thousand tweets. Some of these were single problems retold over a number of tweets, some a retelling of the same problem. But given the size of the UK trans community, this was significant.

Later analysis by trans campaigner Helen Belcher revealed that complaints about GP practices (either about GPs themselves, or other staff in the practice) were far and away the largest category. In addition, over half the complaints about GPs and gender-related services were to do with a refusal to treat or refer, something that at face value is in complete defiance of the GMC's own Good Medical Practice Guide.

Did the author of that *Guardian* piece reminding GPs of the dangers of getting involved in areas where they lack specialist expertise, and the risk of being sued, have a point? The opposite seems to be the case, as the actual consequence for GPs getting it wrong for trans patients is not that great.

There are a number of reasons why this might be the case. To begin with, trans people are highly dependent on the goodwill of a relatively small number of practitioners within a closely knit community of gender specialists. So until they are at least post-op, there are significant dangers to complaining.

One trans patient observed: 'I never complained about my abusive psych because I didn't want to end the only NHS route out.' Another identified a specialist who had stopped anyone else trying to treat them; they had made a formal complaint asking for that specialist no longer to be involved in their care. Yet another tells of attempting to complain and having their next appointment cancelled.

The bottom line: patient after patient spoke of how terrified they were of talking about their experiences because they feared their treatment would be withdrawn. That is an unhealthy situation for just one patient to be in. When that applies across the board to patients seeking assistance in respect of a particular specialism, it is a disgrace.

Even so, the likelihood of anything being done about that situation is negligible. As news of #TransDocFail hit national media, the General Medical Council was forced to admit that it does not carry out Equality Impact Assessments on the origin of complaints about medical practitioners. In other words, they did not monitor complaints by minority group. They were therefore unable to check whether any specific group was suffering from systemic poor practice by GPs – or indeed, any other medical practitioners.

For a while, they assured the trans community they would do better. Helen Belcher worked with complainants to provide a dossier for the GMC to investigate. In the end there were almost 200 substantive complaints that, it was felt, would bear investigation.

Yet over a period of months, these were whittled down and

down again. Perhaps a third of that number, the GMC felt, fitted their own complaints criteria. And then of these, the evidence was contradictory, or denied, or too late. In the end, the hundreds of complaints raised by the trans community, simply vanished like morning mist. Nor is there any evidence, from conversations within the community, of many individuals being prepared to trust the GMC sufficiently to submit formal complaints.

And while the GMC were keen to express their concern and their desire to be supportive of the trans community, in 2017 – four years after #TransDocFail – there is a guide for lesbian, gay and bisexual patients wishing to lodge a complaint, but still no such guide exists for trans patients.

A cynic might imagine that this was, after all, just a very British way of dealing with complaints. Spin it out, salami slice, dismiss one here, another there, on a technicality. Keep expressing sympathy for the victims. In the end, what should have been a wake-up call for the medical profession simply fades away.

If GPs are not at risk from an 'angry trans community', who is?

As noted in 'Prelude: Mapping the World of Trans', there has long been tension between the trans community and the medical profession. The latter is seen not only as gate-keeping access to desperately needed gender services, but also as jealously guarding its central role in the gender identity mix. Two – perhaps three – key issues need to be taken into account in this respect.

The first is that, while the trans community may have ongoing issues with GPs, historically the focus of a much finer ire has been the gender identity clinics themselves.

One trans individual decided, for the sake of their own mental health that they were better off spending money on having surgery done privately. This followed an appalling experience at one gender identity clinic. They were called out in their 'dead name' in the waiting room. The clinician who saw them balked at using the name they had now been known by for many years, eventually giving in only with ill grace. The same clinician then spent the hour of their first interview bullying them and finally ended up with a veiled threat to take them off hormones. At the end of that encounter, the individual was left upset, tearful and, for perhaps the first and only time in their lives, suicidal.

Eventually, they received an apology courtesy of one of the administrative managers of the clinic. The clinician who saw them never bothered to contact them again.

That is one story, but it is repeated time and time again. Trans individuals report bullying, intimidation and manipulation on the part of clinicians. Yet if the only avenue open to them is the NHS, they have no alternative but to swallow their pride and return for more of the same.

It would be unfair to suggest that gender identity clinics are universally like this. Against these tales of woe are to be found many, many satisfied customers: people who will admit, privately, that without the intervention of a GIC they might not be alive today. Also, one major source of discontent appears to have little to do with the specialists themselves, more to do with a toxic interaction of policy and administrative incompetence.

That is, while many trans people are desperate to transition, a proportion vacillate: they want to; they don't want to. So they may book themselves in to a GIC one day – and then, when the time for their appointment comes round, they have changed their mind, but told no one. Given the lengthy waiting lists for all GICs the policy operated is therefore simple: one strike and you're out.

Fail to turn up for an appointment without good reason and you are no longer on the GIC's books. This is outwardly sensible. The issue – a constant with GICs – is that communications get lost or not sent, or otherwise go astray. As a result, far too many patients find that after waiting months for an appointment, the first they hear from a GIC is a letter telling them they have failed to show and are no longer a patient!

The second key issue that affects a significant proportion of GIC patients is the 'dared-to-go-private' hurdle. If, while waiting for an appointment, a trans individual decides to reduce their personal dysphoria by seeking treatment through a private consultant, there may be consequences. Certainly, any hormones they have been prescribed are likely to be stopped once they start at a GIC.

This is, the GICs argue, so as to obtain an untainted base line reading for endocrinological purposes. Many trans people suspect a slightly darker motive: that this is to ensure both dependence on the GIC and control of the individual's pathway through the transition process.

Worse, there have been instances of individuals sent to the back of the queue for daring to take this awful contrary stance and seeking to lessen their distress. One individual, posting to the #TransDocFail campaign told how they had obtained a private diagnosis. Later, after some years on HRT, they wanted to access surgery through the NHS. In WPATH terms, they were already at a point – beyond a point – where surgery should have been permissible. But as far as their GIC was concerned, they should go back to square one. They should stop the HRT, undergo psych assessment, and essentially add at least a couple of years to their waiting time.

They are far from alone. In fact, this experience, of being pushed back is widespread amongst the trans community. The gender establishment does not approve of private practice.

This compounds other problems. In the next section are details of a case begun against trans-supporting GP Dr Helen Webberley. While under investigation, she writes, she cannot treat transgender patients without supervision. But: 'The irony is that the only people appropriate to act in the capacity of supervisor would be the doctors at the Tavistock and Portman Clinic, the very same doctors who have made the complaints against me; and therein lies the rub.'

There is no suggestion of impropriety here. Rather, it is the sense that in a system that is in flux, there should be more input from the trans community. They are, after all, the raison d'être for this entire branch of medicine. 'Nothing about us without us' is a slogan claimed by many groups within the NHS, and endorsed by at least one recent Health Secretary. Yet the actual practice seems to be almost completely the opposite.

The trans community has experienced decades of a medical establishment that talks the good talk, while steadfastly refusing to adapt to patient needs. Those used to dealing with the NHS are all too used to polite spin masquerading as genuine concern. Which is why, for all the superficial reasonableness, many in the community will view yet another piece – this time in *The Guardian* – arguing that the trans community deserves better, but that GPs are worried about the risk of litigation, as fundamentally insulting.

Trans-positive practitioners singled out

A number of recent events colour the trans view of the medical profession, and go some way to explain the fury unleashed in the #TransDocFail project. Because in the last 15 years, there have been two – now three – high-profile cases brought before the GMC in which individual practitioners were accused of malpractice in respect of their treatment of trans patients.

Not one of them reflects the mass of complaints documented here. Each represented an attack on practitioners felt to be trans-positive in their approach to treatment. Each has therefore been interpreted by the trans community as an attempt by the status quo to control and ration healthcare for trans patients.

In 2006–2007, Russell Reid, a consultant psychiatrist specialising in the treatment of trans individuals was hauled before the General Medical Council on charges of serious professional misconduct. This arose following complaints brought by doctors working at the Charing Cross Gender Identity Clinic as well as some of his former patients. It was alleged that he had breached international standards of care (at that time, the Harry Benjamin Standards) by inappropriately prescribing cross-gender hormones to patients and referring them for sex re-assignment surgery without carrying out adequate assessment.

According to trans lobbying group, Press for Change, Reid received support from more than 150 patients as well as a number of experts in the area. Hundreds more patients posted positive comments during and after the hearing. In the end, Reid was found guilty of serious professional misconduct, primarily for failing to communicate fully with patient GPs and for insufficiently documenting his reasons for departing from the Benjamin Standards. However, the panel 'determined that it would be in the public interest as well as your own interests if you were to return to practice under strict conditions'. It then allowed him to return to practice, subject to some restrictions on his practice and hormone prescriptions for the next 12 months.

This attracted a certain amount of (sensational) press interest at the time. Much of it came from individuals identified in Chapter 1 as trans-sceptic or outright anti-trans, who justified their interest in terms of being in support of trans people.

The event that kicked off the #TransDocFail campaign was remarkably similar. In 2012/13, the news broke that the GMC were again investigating a practitioner, Dr Richard Curtis of TransHealth, in respect of allegations of malpractice in treating trans patients.

Dr Curtis was no saint. Equally, he made available one of the few pathways to trans treatment that did not wind through the uncertain straits of the NHS. The mere fact that he was out there doing what he did provided a certain hope to the community and reassurance that an alternative existed.

Complaints were in relation to the alleged inappropriate administering of sex-change hormones to patients. In most instances this was a technical omission, in the sense that he failed to conform to UK protocols for treatment, using prescription of oestrogen as a diagnostic tool, rather than delay prescribing as is the norm in UK clinics (but not everywhere in the rest of the world). It was also alleged he had made an unsuitable referral for gender re-assignment surgery. Once again, practitioners from existing GICs were involved in the complaints, and once again, the same trans-sceptic elements were out in the press expressing their concern that trans patients should only receive the best.

And as documented above, the furious response of the trans community was made known to the GMC. It is not that the trans community does not care about malpractice. Rather it is disgust at the complete lack of even-handedness in those supposedly regulating the medical community. There is concern, too, at the hypocrisy of a press that can ignore mistreatment of trans individuals for years, but instantly reach for the outrage mode when someone is discovered to be treating trans people the way they would wish to be treated.

In 2015, the GMC dropped all charges and Dr Curtis was given the green light to continue to practise. But – perhaps overwhelmed by the stress of this ordeal – two years later, in 2017, he announced that he would be closing his practice.

And now, as 2017 draws to a close, the GMC is once more investigating a practitioner who has proven a godsend to many in the trans community. Once more, standards and prescribing are under discussion. Once more, the gender identity experts are to the fore in bringing complaints, and, to the rear, the press is salivating at the prospect of a juicy scandal.

This is the case of Dr Helen Webberley, a GP based now in Wales. Her work with transgender health started when she worked as a transgender specialist in Worcester and as a communication skills educator at the University of Birmingham. In 2005 she transferred to Wales and took up a partnership in a GP practice.

It was while working with a trans group in Worcester that she encountered her first trans patient. Discussing treatment options, it quickly became clear that London, the only option available to Welsh GPs, was impractical and effectively impossible for the patient to access. So she took the unusual step of prescribing HRT directly.

From small beginnings, over a two-year period, she dealt with 3000 enquiries for advice and information. To begin she treated around 550 individuals – although not all of these were prescribed hormones. Rather, she claims, her aim is to match treatment to patient needs: sometimes counselling, sometimes hormones and, in some instances referring onward for surgical intervention. She has, however, been criticised by the medical establishment for various reasons:

- The fact that she offers online consultation and diagnosis. This, it is claimed, makes it impossible to establish the full patient–practitioner relationship.
- The age at which she is prepared to prescribe certain treatments. This includes the provision of hormones at age 12 (in one instance) and a willingness to prescribe puberty blockers without the year-long wait.
- A number of technical issues around prescribing practice.

In respect of the first, this is an odd criticism. The NHS is already trialling the use of online consultation. Where physical examination is required a face-to-face consultation will still be necessary. But it is likely that this approach will increasingly be commonplace in rural areas, such as those where Webberley is based, as well as areas where access to GPs is limited. It also addresses an issue regularly raised by trans patients: that with so few GICs based in a restricted number of locations, simply attending for assessment and treatment is a major barrier to those on low incomes wishing to transition.

For the second, she freely admits to being out of line with UK guidelines on hormones, but cites a growing consensus around this approach in other parts of the world, including the US and the Netherlands. She questions the rigid age limits set by UK clinics and makes an argument based on two key principles.

- Harm: If the limits do more harm than good, in terms of increased risks of depression and suicide, then continuing to enforce them is in direct conflict with the principle to which most practitioners are signed 'do no harm'.
- Competence: The Gillick principle suggests that where a child is competent to take a medical decision, then they are entitled to do so. Webberley argues that if a child is competent to make a decision on hormones, it is possibly unlawful to refuse their request.

Beyond this, Webberley is a strong advocate of rooting trans healthcare more firmly in general practice and consigning the current costly, bureaucratic model to the dustbin of history. This, she has claimed, is far more cost-effective than the alternatives, as well as far more humane. It is also closely aligned to what the NHS, by way of a consultation circulating in 2017, would like to happen.

Why don't more GPs take this route? As already seen, there is clearly a reluctance on the part of GPs to take on this responsibility. According to Webberley, it is 'a mix of lack of knowledge and fear of the current gender establishment'. Webberley herself tells of a patient to whom she was prescribing hormones who was discharged from Charing Cross GIC for the heinous crime of being prescribed hormones by her. In a further move unlikely to assist this individual's mental health, she claims that Charing Cross then contacted the patient's local GP to demand they stop hormones.

Despite this, there is no reason for any GP not to follow in Webberley's footsteps. Transgender treatment is not covered in standard training for endocrinology or in psychiatry. The core skills are not hard to acquire. To this end, Webberley has been heavily involved in GP training that aims to raise knowledge in this area, as well as working to promote a GP-based model for trans healthcare.

This last has already born some fruit with NHS Wales now showing a far greater readiness to listen to and learn from the trans community.

For now – late 2017 – the case against Webberley is still to proceed. As before, how the GMC deals with it will be watched closely by the trans community. However, what is actually happening in respect of the treatment of trans individuals is, courtesy of that 2017 consultation, now a matter of high medical politics.

GPs, as a body, are resistant to taking on responsibility for trans healthcare – and that resistance is growing, to the point where practices such as taking on prescriptions from GICs are, in some parts of the country, seriously at risk. A few are interested in setting up specialist support groups, and this, rather than making every GP an expert in trans healthcare, may be the way to go.

In the meantime, those that do provide this support are often driven to do so privately – to charge for their services – because there is no framework within the NHS into which they fit.

This, though, is resisted by the GICs, which continue to wage covert war on private practitioners by means of the GMC and jealously guard their role as gate-keepers to trans healthcare nationwide. Although the NHS consultation is strong on advocating a role for GPs it also includes provision that access to some NHS services, such as gender re-assignment surgery, *must* be through GICs.

This is fine, if surgery is de-coupled from other treatments, such as hormones. If it is not, then this creates a dilemma – again – for trans patients desperate for treatment, and pushes them, once more, back towards private practice and self-medding – with the added twist that if they admit to the latter, they may find themselves refused NHS treatment.

Failing Syn: the NHS in action

The NHS system has defeated many trans people over the years, including some far more expert in dealing with systemic intransigence than Syn. For, though Syn was good at doing her research and working out how something *should* work, she lacked the practical skills necessary to make things happen in the face of inertia and rejection.

To begin with, she attended a private consultation (at her own expense) in May 2012 with Dr Michael Perring, a psychotherapist with extensive experience of dealing with transgender patients. Dr Perring provided a standard diagnosis, in conformity with the WPATH guidelines, which evaluated Synestra as a 'well-adjusted self-medicating transgender person'.

He also provided guidelines for her NHS GP to follow in terms of medication and blood tests that Synestra would need. The latter was communicated the same month by letter to Syn's GP, then located in a GP practice in north London. Syn's parents have been unable to find any correspondence from this period. However, as they understand it, this was chased up, again by letter, following a second consultation with Perring in June.

It is possible – more than possible – that the rejection was verbal or simply not recorded officially. However, their understanding is that Syn was rejected at this time because Perring was 'not on the right panel for the budget area'.

In fact – and in hindsight – Syn had simply failed to understand how the system worked. As described above, GPs may treat trans patients who arrive with a private diagnosis, but they are not required to. In other words, Syn had a diagnosis, but because it came from the wrong place, that permitted her GP to treat her as though she did not have one.

In piecing this story together, the individual that Syn most likely dealt with at the time was contacted. In addition to warning us that any inaccuracy would be dealt with in the strictest of terms(!), they made clear both that they were equal opps in terms of how they treated trans patients, and that they would *not* initiate treatment of trans patients who came through a non-NHS pathway.

Synestra's letter from Dr Perring therefore got her nowhere.

It is possible – we can only now surmise – that Syn hoped, by seeing an independent consultant, that she could shortcut her way to prescription drugs and an endocrinologist. This was not an entirely unreasonable proposition. What she likely did not know is that as far as treatment of trans individuals is concerned, large parts of north London are notoriously poor.

Even if a GP is unable to prescribe the hormones requested by a patient, they can make out a referral to a GP who can. They can, and should, also begin the process of referring the patient to a gender identity clinic. It is clear that neither of these things happened. Why not? Family and friends suspect two factors in play.

The first is that famous Syn reluctance to make a fuss. The GP turned her down. So rather than demand her rights to treatment, she went away. The second – and this again goes to the fact that in 2012 she had not had much contact with the wider trans community

– she was not talking to people with experience of the system, who knew what to expect, who could have guided her.

Nothing much happened now for another six months or so. This, too, was typical of Syn: rebuffed, she would go away to lick her wounds, build up the confidence to try again. In this period she moved first to Lewisham and then, off and on, back to Stevenage, with her parents. Like many another student, it was not entirely clear where her 'primary abode' was for official purposes. Some weeks it was Lewisham. Other weeks it was Stevenage.

In early 2013, and at the prompting of her parents, she approached a Stevenage practice. She got Dr Perring to write a letter. That did not go well. Her GP agreed to blood tests, but not to prescribing. He declared she did not live sufficiently in Stevenage to qualify as a local patient, removed her from the practice list and told her to go and register with a GP in London.

Purely anecdotal evidence suggests that this pickiness as to where patients lived appears not to have extended to non-trans residents. A local from Letchworth tells of an incident, a few years back, when her daughter was staying over in Stevenage for a few days and was taken in to this practice for a minor medical problem. Without asking her permission, the practice simply moved her daughter's registration – not even signing her up as a temporary patient. When she next sought treatment at her local (Letchworth) practice, she was shocked to find her daughter no longer registered there and not entitled to be treated locally.

Unfortunately, Syn made it clear that she wanted to be in control of the process, so her parents got on with life as usual believing that the ball was now rolling. This was compounded by the fact that any time they asked, Syn simply told them it was in the hands of her GP. For most of 2013, she did not even mention that she had been removed from the practice list. This left her largely unsupported in other respects, including her drug issues, which were now becoming more serious. There is no evidence that she signed up with any other practice, although her parents believe that she attempted to sign up in London a couple of times, without success. They conclude that for at least a year she was effectively without a GP.

In 2014 Synestra was starting to show signs of frustration. Her parents asked what was wrong and she explained the issues with the local GP. Amanda was livid, especially as, by that time, Syn was very clearly living in Stevenage for much of the time. She persuaded Syn to make a joint appointment and her father went with her. Finally, the practice agreed to take her on as a patient and the question of getting Syn seen for gender re-assignment was raised.

There were issues over Syn's private consultation, which the practice claimed never to have received. Besides, they were unwilling to take any notice of this consultation because Dr Perring was 'not on the correct panel', so they could do nothing about it. In fact, according to Synestra's parents, they managed to lose the Perring letter twice! They therefore hand-delivered a copy.

The practice also informed Syn that they first needed a psychological report based on a local assessment and would then decide on hormone treatment. However, as noted above, this was not strictly necessary, given the assessment by Dr Perring. No mention was made of a referral to a GIC. They appeared unaware that by 2014 the requirement for a local assessment had been removed, and they were entitled to refer Synestra directly.

Even with this intervention, nothing happened. 2014 passed, apparently without any reference to the GIC. Syn's parents say they have lost track of the excuses. On their next visit, the GP claimed that a referral to the GIC had definitely been sent in late 2014, although they are not sure this ever happened.

A part of the problem, according to Sonny, a local decorator who also works with local LGBT organisations to provide support to individuals, who helped Synestra that year, is that by now the recreational drugs were taking their toll. Syn, never the most organised of individuals, was even more disorganised. It is possible, Sonny believes, that Syn may have missed key appointments, but it is difficult to be sure.

In the end, it was Sonny putting his foot down that did the trick. He felt that she just needed a referral and, he explains, 'the story of her not getting one was just winding me up'. Worried that Syn was not receiving adequate treatment for a range of complex interlocking issues, he attended the practice with her in January 2015. As Sonny remembers it, the GP claimed he needed to obtain blood tests for her first. This is not required in the NHS pathway; in fact, GICs often reject blood tests carried out by GPs, preferring that such tests be carried out through their own facilities.

Sonny, however, insisted that blood tests were unnecessary. He suggested that since the GP appointment was short, the most useful thing to do would be to get a referral off while he and Syn were present. He stood over the GP, filling in blanks for him, in the necessary referral document. The entire process, which Syn had been waiting for for over two years took just five minutes.

The referral was made, although a subsequent response suggests that it was not actually put in the post until 9 February 2015.

The story, like so many stories highlighted under the #TransDocFail banner, combines mismanagement with complacency. They ask: Would medical professionals treat any other category of patient with such disdain? Would any other patient have needed, as Synestra did, to fight every inch of her journey – or take three years in working their way through the system?

In June 2015, the Stevenage practice convened a meeting, at which it was finally agreed that they would provide Synestra with the medication first prescribed for her in 2012. According to her father, he only became aware of this decision the week before Synestra's funeral.

In August 2015, notification came through from Charing Cross GIC to say that they were happy to accept Syn for treatment. But by then, it was too late. Synestra was already dead – had died a week earlier.

CHAPTER 5

Into the Darkness

Decline

After the heady days of north London, what followed, even if more of the same, was always going to be anti-climax. That seems to have been the case with Synestra, who now alternated London and Stevenage, together with a drug problem that for most of the time just got worse.

It also seems to have been a time when Syn's flaws began to dominate. Outwardly, as all bore witness, she had an outlandish character that made her look very confident to a stranger. Inside, though, the Syn that few ever really saw was exceptionally shy. Her last boyfriend, Joey, talks of this. So, too, does close friend Dani, who adds: 'Very few people ever really knew her. She just fed people an illusion of the character she had created.'

She was also 'forever alienated by her own intelligence'. As Dani, again, puts it: 'Syn was insanely intelligent to the point where you'd almost not want to say stuff around her. At the same time, she was totally arrogant: she was the best, and she knew it. She was the best sex worker in her game and she was proud of that. She felt that there was not one person in the world who could tell her what she didn't know.'

Yet alongside this intelligence was something else: a complete lack of 'street savvy'. Syn seemed to enjoy risk. Or perhaps she just didn't understand it. On one occasion, after Dani's club closed, a security team member came down to tell her that her friend looked like she was in trouble. Dani went outside, to find Syn in lingerie and 9″ heels, surrounded by a gang of young men, telling them to fuck off. She had absolutely no concept of the danger she was in.

Another time, she was leaving the club with, according to Dani, 'some very dodgy bloke'. Dani suggested she would be safer not to go. Syn shrugged. Yes she was.

Syn's first stop, after north London, was Lewisham, where she lived for a little under a year, from late 2012 to June 2013. Once more, Syn shared with close friends. At various times, there were three, sometimes four individuals living there, including Syn.

Yet Lewisham was not the best of places for her, as it was in Lewisham that bad things multiplied. On one occasion she fell out with a girl also living there. She accused Syn of making a play for her boyfriend. Syn hadn't, but had introduced him to another girl, so she hit Syn with a wine bottle. Syn spent a couple of days injured and in bed. She was concussed and in need of medical attention. But she preferred not to make a fuss. Later, explaining why she had not pressed charges, she said it wasn't the girl's fault.

This passive, fatalistic, reaction was increasingly typical of Syn. In 2013/14 she arrived at Dani's house, looking beaten and dishevelled. She had gone to see a client in a hotel and had been attacked and raped by a number of men. Dani wanted to call the police. Syn said, 'No – they aren't there for people like me.'

Dani felt, as always, that there was little she or anyone could do to help...and Syn used the shower, got fully glammed up and went on to her next client.

It was also while in Lewisham that Syn had around £12,000 stolen, as well as a very expensive pair of boots. Again, Syn did little about it, beyond suspecting everyone and no one. According to her boyfriend Ben, she was starting to get paranoid, and suspected everyone except him – and then only because she said he was a very bad liar.

This, her father remembers, hit her very hard, and it was around this point that they began to be concerned that Syn was becoming depressed. She was at home sitting in the family lounge when she opened up to him about this. She broke down crying: not for the money itself, but for what it represented, a major stop along the way to her transition. And this loss would set her back months.

This period coincides with the beginning of the first of two significant relationships in Syn's life. The first was with Ben, around four years her senior.

They had friends in common. An important bridge from Syn to Ben was Wayne, who lived in the Lewisham flat and was a close friend and confidant. Syn and Ben met in March 2013 and initially, it seems, Syn disliked because him because he was 'besotted' and 'drove her mad'.

This Ben freely owns up to. On first meeting he was taken with her physically: her style, her 'beautiful long black hair' and her 'insane heels'. He was also seriously attracted by her intellect, and the fact she was not constrained by cultural norms: 'She talked openly, honestly about stuff in a way that no one else had.' He had never met anyone so honest.

Whatever their initial doubts, they clicked. On that first night, they went back to Ben's place and just talked. She was, Ben admits, all he could think about for week, and in the end that feeling was mutual. Their relationship began that same month; and in April, Ben moved into Lewisham with Syn.

It seems fair to suggest that Ben and Syn were bad for one another, and both knew it. Both were drug users when they met, but Ben more closely fitted the profile of an addict. Syn was more experienced when it came to sex work, and she suggested that Ben have a go as well. He did, admitting that he felt his eyes had been thoroughly opened by Syn, though he only ever earned about half what Syn did!

Yet it was not just Ben who was addicted to Syn: she, too, quickly developed an equal passion for him.

They started off going out a lot, but ended up staying in, with just one another for company. Perhaps aware of the dangers inherent in the situation, she ended the relationship in June.

It was circumstance that brought them back together again. A few weeks after Ben left Lewisham, Syn was abducted by two people in Soho. They fed her a cocktail of drugs in the back of a car and took her back to their squat, where they held her for some hours before she escaped.

This incident got her talking to Ben again, and in September 2013 they were back together, though now Ben was living in King's Cross. This 'second bite' at a relationship lasted until March 2014, when Ben overdosed and went into rehab. It was around this time that she and Ben made their one and only foray into online porn: a home-shot short featuring the two of them. For a while, according to Ben, this made good money online. Then it was ripped off by commercial porn providers and they lost control of it.

The last straw was when her father's cousin visited from the US in June 2013. It was Syn's 21st birthday. Amanda, John and cousin dropped by to pick Syn up, unannounced – and walked in on a sex orgy in full fling. Never mind the orgy; they were also not impressed by the fact that the flat was filthy. Knees and shoes would stick to the carpet, and there was rat poison under the bed. Enough, they decided was enough, and paid to move Syn out and into Barnet with her boyfriend. She lasted in her first flat for a short while and was in the second place for about a month, when parents again suggested she move.

What followed was the stuff of nightmare for every parent, as Syn increasingly oscillated between London and Stevenage. After a serious incident, Ben went into rehab from March 2014 to June 2014, and both he and Syn were back in their respective parental homes.

In the first half of 2014, she dropped out of college – again – this time pleading that she was ill and desperately needed a year to get her head back together. Officially, she took a year off from September 2014.

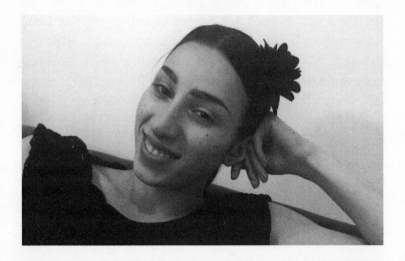

So she was back home – but this was not ideal either. Friends attest that the drugs were taking a toll. John and Amanda tell of doors being left open, music being on at all hours, pans being placed on the hob and left to boil dry. The front door was left open and the dog went wandering the streets early one morning. After that, they took away her key. Superglue all over the carpet! A broken glass tray; obviously trying to clear the mess up, Syn walked all over the glass in bare feet. Almost 'teenage stuff', but it felt like Syn, already notoriously scatter-brained, was becoming even more disorganised.

One time, her father took her into town to fetch some tablets: she went into the wrong shop. Walking back, she got into the wrong car and, apparently, startled the man sitting in it by explaining to him, matter-of-factly: 'You're not my dad.'

Email exchanges from this period, between Syn and her mother, highlight the sheer frustration of attempting to support a child who was out of control.

Ben owns, later, to being afraid for her all the time when they were together. She'd go out and not answer her phone for a couple of days, and that would 'drive him nuts'. Most of the time she would be fine, but sometimes something had happened. Even then, most things were 'not a problem', as far as Syn was concerned.

Yet there was a far darker side to this, too. Syn's parents were concerned that she made the place more vulnerable: drug dealers came to the house at all hours. Syn still carried on some sex work, and on more than one occasion was picked up by punters in front of the house. She was robbed again: and again she lost several thousand pounds in cash.

Her parents were then victims of an aggravated burglary: masked robbers entered the house and stole a large amount of cash. At knifepoint. Their suspicion is that they followed Syn home and into the house in order to obtain money for drugs that Syn had not paid for.

When challenged on her drug use, she became aggressive, dismissing her parents as 'old fogies', who understood 'nothing about drugs or the situation'. Around this time, too, she was on her blog, dismissing anyone who dared to criticise her drug habits. In response to one, she wrote: 'I don't care if ignorant people like you condemn me... I know I am right and your attempts to bring me down smash on my narcissistic armour!'

It felt like her earlier arrogance, fuelled by drug side-effects, was now in overdrive – and Syn was out of control and on a path to self-destruct.

Ben talks of her becoming increasingly paranoid. She would talk of friends plotting against her. One time she accused Ben of stealing her etizolam. He told her: 'I haven't got it. Why don't you look in the chest of drawers behind you?' Syn looked and found it exactly where Ben had suggested. Her response: 'You must have thrown it while we were talking.' These symptoms got markedly more serious when she was not sleeping. A part of her drug habit was now directed simply towards getting her a night's sleep.

Matters went from bad to worse in mid-2014, with an episode that resulted in Syn being officially excluded from her parents' home for over a month. She was due in Marbella in August for her facial feminisation surgery. Initially, she had been planning to go on her own or perhaps find a friend to go with her. Amanda argued that this was a major surgical procedure: she would be in hospital for days, and in need of extensive support after. She would need a 'plan B'. In the end, Syn agreed, and the two were due to fly out to Marbella on Thursday 31 July.

Two days before, there was an episode that shattered this temporary harmony. Syn's relationship with her brother, Adam, had been growing more prickly, alternating love and support with sibling rivalry. Amanda had packed up for the evening, and Syn was in Adam's room, 'showing him how to accomplish something on the computer'.

By morning, though, something had happened: Adam was lying in an empty bath, flailing, his face contorted. Syn said she thought he had taken something. An ambulance was called and Adam was rushed to hospital. He clearly had taken something. The suspicion, never confirmed, was that Syn had dropped some GBL into his Lucozade – though why was never adequately explained.

When the ambulance arrived, Syn was quick to explain that she had given him something to bring him out of whatever state he was in. The ambulance driver concurred. It was a good idea, but since the tablet Syn had obtained was off the internet, Syn could have no idea what was in it and therefore no idea whether her actions made things worse or better.

Once at the hospital, Syn continued to be critical, saying they did not know what they were doing. It is likely that she and Ben did have a better idea of how to treat a drugs overdose, from personal experience. The hospital seemed less than eager to treat someone they saw as simply another addict. In light of what happened to Syn less than a year later, there is a particular irony to this observation.

With Adam responding well to treatment, Syn and her mother flew out to Marbella the next day for Syn's surgery. They returned 14 days later to find armed police waiting for them on the tarmac: the arms, it seems, were because airport police are routinely armed, and not because they expected any serious resistance. Syn was arrested, both were taken through customs, and their bags were searched. Syn spent the night at Hatfield in the cells.

Because Adam was still technically a child, social services were involved. On her release, Syn was barred from returning to the family home. In the end, Adam refused to press charges against his sister. No further action was taken, beyond a visit from a detective sergeant who came to discuss drugs with Syn. As was her wont, Syn attempted to argue that she knew what she was doing and that the drugs could not harm her.

For once, though, she had met her match, and the police officer put her thoroughly in her place.

By now, Syn's drug habit had progressed from recreational drug user to addict, both physical and mental. The signs were all around: post-op, for instance, in Marbella, Syn happily took all the morphine on offer and then demanded more. She was quite capable of taking a dose that the attending medics warned was dangerous.

There are some dissenting voices amongst those who knew her in her early partying days. Dani, for instance, remembers her as having an enormous capacity for taking drugs. She said: 'I have never seen someone take so much, or with such tolerance. She could out-party anyone, take massive doses of MDMA, ketamine, whatever – and she would never look like she was on drugs. Friends talked of her as invincible. But obviously that was her downfall.'

Ben too remarked at this point that Syn's dependence on drugs might put her life in danger. On occasion, when she took too much GHB she would lose consciousness, even stop breathing. Yet, as far as Syn was concerned, this was not an issue. On one occasion Ben called an ambulance. She was angry as she really could not see what all the bother was about. The next time she wasn't breathing properly, Ben filmed it on the phone for when she woke up. Her response: she refused to believe what was on the video, and claimed that the phone mic was not picking up her breath.

Syn was at least now talking to support workers about the possibility that she might have issues with drugs. This was how she first met Sonny, the LGBT support worker who would later help her with her application to the GIC. In June 2014, Sonny was working with the Viewpoint mental health charity. Shortly before that, Amanda met with Sonny and told him that her daughter was trans and using drugs.

Sonny's first concern was to get Syn off drugs, and he recommended she access the Living Room, a local treatment centre in Stevenage. Syn agreed to meet – but she was more focused on getting her referral to Charing Cross. She told Sonny she had been on the case for over two years, and the NHS were monumentally unhelpful.

It was Sonny, too, who now agreed, after the incident with Adam, to put her up in his home, in Welwyn Garden City for around six weeks. This lasted for a month or so until it was clear that Syn and Ben were back together again. Rather than becoming a safe haven for Syn, there was a danger that Sonny's home would turn into a place where Syn and Ben could rekindle their addiction.

So once more Syn was out. She was still officially barred from her family home, so her parents took her to her grandparents in Barkston. Syn made an effort, and, by the time she did return, she appeared in better health than she had been for many months. She and Ben now found a place, once more in Barnet, from which they were evicted shortly before Christmas, allegedly for being too noisy. Ben, though, suspects because the owner's son had developed a dislike for Syn.

And then, in February 2015, Ben decided he couldn't do it any more, because it was clear to him that they fed off each other. Ben needed to stay clean, drug-free, but living with Syn, both were moving deeper into drugs, including heavier substances such as crystal meth.

So Ben moved out and Syn moved back to Stevenage once more.

Looking up

2014 may have looked thoroughly bleak as far as Syn was concerned. But 2015, despite a number of ups and downs, was a year when things finally started to go right. To start with, there was the referral to the GIC: no sign yet that anything would come of that; but following her visit to her GP with Sonny in January, it finally looked as though that might start to come good.

Small things. Official things. A new passport; and, in April, Amanda dropped her a line to say 'told you so': 'You now have a new NHS number as a female. You also have a new birth certificate in the name of Synestra.'

And then two dramatic events that looked set to change her life for good. At Easter, Syn was at home in Stevenage and acting strangely. At that time, her parents were unaware of the effects – and the side-effects – of GHB. In desperation, they threw away her GHB stash. Syn went into withdrawal. An ambulance was called and Syn was rushed to hospital. In the end, she needed to be detoxed in hospital, and John and Amanda remember that as a terrible time: Syn had the shakes, was paranoid, and felt she might die. In desperation, they contacted Ben for advice – as someone who had been through this himself they felt he might have sensible advice to give – and he advised hospital to give her Valium.

This, though, seemed to act as wake-up call. Syn finally agreed she had a problem, finally agreed to do rehab. She signed on with local drug dependency service, Spectrum, who prescribed medication for her mental health and dependency issues. John was on hand to chaperone and care for her, as well as make sure she stuck with substitute/prescription drugs. To begin with, these were locked away in John's office, to prevent Syn overdosing on the substitutes. Yet, after a few days she began to adapt.

Of course, there was one final twist from her Stevenage GP. Spectrum wrote to them explaining what support Syn needed, and when Syn's parents chased this up they were told – yet again – that they hadn't received any correspondence. Yet again, a letter was hand-delivered, with fingers crossed that the delay had not created further problems for her.

Then Syn found romance again. Shortly after she started the rehab programme, she was 'clean', and the old Syn started to return. Chatting to her father one evening she said she felt lonely. John suggested she make a list of friends, and then split that list into people who would give her drugs and those who wouldn't and then get in touch with the second.

The first name on that list was Joey, a friend of a friend. Syn contacted him through WhatsApp, and not long after they arranged to go out to eat. John remembers that night well: she spent for ever getting ready, and then she came down wearing a dress and she looked absolutely stunning. Joey was knocked over the moment he met her. It was, he says, 'an amazing night I will never forget'. Syn had messaged him earlier in the day saying that she was going to look glamorous, and he had better look smart.

When he first saw her, 'Syn really did take my breath away. Her jet-black hair streaked with gold, her 7-inch red heels with cute little pink socks and a flowing white dress that perfectly cloaked her model-esque body.'

Over drinks, Syn started on what Joey described as a university-level science examination. This was not to catch him out so much as size him up.

That was Syn. She didn't want to have conversations about mundanities. She had a fierce intensity and a passion for what she was interested in. Yet she was always open to new ideas and conclusions if they could reach her razor-sharp intellect.

They spent the evening talking and, when Syn came home that night she told her father: 'I think I'm in love.' What about the rest of the list? Oh, you can forget that!

The feeling seemed to be mutual. Over the next few months they almost but didn't quite move in together. When Joey asked why she didn't just move some clothes down to his place in Putney, she turned, throwing her hair sideways, and said: 'I'm Synestra De Courcy.' She was ever the perfectionist!

Joey worked hard to satisfy Syn's culinary desires. In between meals, Syn would beat him, time and time again, on Mortal Kombat. They were proposing to move to a flat in Finsbury Park and planning out the rest of their lives together. They became inseparable; and Syn was shaping up, staying clean!

Joe was, in almost every way, chalk to Ben's cheese: as someone not so closely associated with Syn's former lifestyle, he gave her a route out from it, as well as a dependable shoulder to lean on. Ben, who confessed to still being in love with Syn, recognised that in her relationship with Joey she felt much more settled.

Life was not entirely without its darker moments, still. In June, she and Joey went clubbing in Vauxhall. Syn was raped, again, in the toilets. She was devastated, although, as she wrote to her mother after the event, not even the second or third time such a thing had happened to her.

Joey, also, felt responsible, telling Syn's parents he had been drunk when they arrived, and subsequently they got separated. He apologised, promised to take better care of Syn in future – and was shocked at not being reprimanded, but instead warned that this was what he was getting into. They were desperate for Joey to take care of her, but they felt he needed to understand her drug-taking history.

Around this time, it seems, she was hatching ideas of returning to YouTube. Not, though to do tutorials, which were everywhere and which, in Syn's view, spoon-fed information and stunted creativity. Rather, she appeared to be thinking of something more akin to a masterclass for make-up people.

She started talking about returning to college; and she was also in discussion with a potential sponsor who was prepared to invest in a new line of cosmetics to be created by Syn.

All, it seemed, was finally coming right. Syn's parents breathed a sigh of relief.

One final party

In late July, Amanda and John remember, Joey and Syn came back to their home for an evening meal. It was, in hindsight, a magic moment: Syn once more, her old self, happy with her new partner.

Her parents were going away the following day to Tenerife. Joey and Syn were invited, but they declined. They planned to party in London that weekend. So with the family abroad, Syn left the family home to meet Joey in London.

She met up with Joey at a club in London on Saturday night (the Wayout Club), and they went on to a house party. From there they went to the home of an acquaintance and continued to talk and socialise. Syn was tired and went into the bedroom to lie down. Around 7pm, one of those present noticed Synestra appeared not to be breathing. An ambulance was called and CPR attempted unsuccessfully – but at 7.18pm on Sunday 26 July she was declared dead.

The coroner returned a verdict of drug-related death. She said: 'It seems to me all the evidence points in the same direction.' An autopsy found traces of mephedrone ('Meow Meow') in her system. Witnesses described how Synestra had been using GBL in the hours before her death. Tragically for Syn, and as pointed out by the coroner, the fact that she had been successfully coming off drugs may have contributed to this outcome. For once you stop taking a particular drug, your tolerance levels drop dramatically. So a dose that previously you tolerated with ease could now prove fatal.

Speaking at the inquest later, Joey said: 'Synestra was one of the most beautiful persons I have ever met. She was warm, highly intelligent, an enigma.'

For Sonny, Syn would in time have been a great role model to the trans community and would have been popular much more widely.

Interviewed for this book, Lux could only add: 'The brightest stars shine the shortest – she was the loveliest, sweetest girl, and the world is at a loss for her not being in it.'

At her funeral, Joey spoke from his heart. He said: 'I genuinely believe that we should live our lives the way Syn would have wanted us to. That's with utter self-belief, to live in the now, to follow our hearts, to be brave enough not to accept anything less than we feel we deserve, but not be selfish and to do right by the people that love us.'

Afterword

The best thing about being a writer and a journalist is the fact that you get the chance to change your mind. Because no matter what the story, big or small, of earth-shattering importance or massively inconsequential, when people let you into their lives, it is a two-way process. Any journalist who claims otherwise is either walled in beyond learning, or comes to the table with a massive agenda.

People change you: by example, by persuasion, by the sheer fact of their living. Whatever you thought you knew at the outset, you discover you are less sure of. Minor details, the small change of everyday living, take on a greater import and inevitably change the way you view the story.

So it is – so it was – with Synestra's story. One half – the personal half – started out as neat moral tale: a parable of incompetence and uncaring. Syn, I imagined, came to the table as supplicant, begging crumbs from a hostile and institutionally transphobic NHS. Syn was failed; and thereafter, all that befell her was 'someone else's fault'.

Apparently abandoned by the NHS, she teetered in and out of depression, a condition that both costs money to treat and could also have been a further bar to her being treated for her gender dysphoria. She determined to self-medicate and to pay for her own surgery: so she set out to do so the only way that many young trans women can, as a sex worker.

She was spending up to £500 some months to obtain hormones

that should have been available for the cost of a simple prescription on the NHS. She was robbed, assaulted and raped. She developed a drug habit, in part as coping mechanism.

All of these, as far as her parents are concerned, are a direct consequence of a failure by the NHS to step up to the modest challenge of dealing with her case and providing her with some hope.

I still believe that, to an extent. There is no excuse for practising GPs to turn away a trans patient, to belittle their issues or to plead systemic issues as reasons for not helping. Although, no surprise, my work over the past few years has taught me to have few good expectations of the NHS in this respect. Because while there are many, many instances of great practice, there is also far too much that is beyond poor. In part, this is the result of systems that have been created, seemingly, for the sole purpose of making the precise location of responsibility invisible. Individuals see this as a brilliant excuse for disguising out-and-out prejudice against trans individuals with a shrug and an 'I'm sorry – there's nothing I can do.'

This effect was very much in play here. People who should have helped Syn did not. Although, people who did not need to help her came through magnificently.

This, though, is to treat Syn as no more than passive subject throughout: the recipient of bad professional behaviour, unable to do more than shrug and bear it. This, I think, now is wrong. Though not entirely so.

For Syn had two traits which, in the final analysis, were to let her down. First, as every trans person who has ever battled their way through the various systems that society has created to embed unchanging gender, you need to fight, and you need to be canny.

Syn was perhaps less of a fighter than she needed to be in her own cause. She could analyse situations to a fine degree, work out for herself how to create complex and unlawful chemical substances and ultimately find her way to people who could help her. She also, it appears, managed to work her way through the Gender Recognition Panel, which is no mean feat in itself. Yet she lacked the particular skill set necessary to work her way through the NHS.

In that she was not the first, and most certainly will not be the last. The NHS defeated her, keeping her, for several long years when she likely needed advice, help, counselling, at arm's length. Only at the very end – and after others had intervened on her behalf – did it grudgingly let her in.

That, you might say, was her own failure – but to do so would be cruel and unreasonable. As cruel, perhaps, as demanding that persons with a badly broken arm fill out several complex forms in their own handwriting before you condescend to treat them. When it comes to obtaining treatment for gender dysphoria, there is, as for so many other specialisms, a postcode lottery.

Yet on top of that there is also something else: the jobsworth test, which states (nowhere formally) that before you can obtain treatment you must leap many hurdles. In some places, you will find the nature of those hurdles and the steps you must take to overcome them explained in great detail. Elsewhere, that information is scarce. Another form of postcode lottery, if you will.

To get through it, you need tenacity: an agility when it comes to dealing with unreasonable bureaucracy. You need to persist. And Syn, for all her intelligence and accomplishments in the academic field was not good at this. She understood what needed to happen, understood outwardly the sorts of steps that she needed to take to arrive at her end; and when doing what she knew she should do failed, she was stumped.

How far this was personal arrogance, how far something else will always be up for debate. Her friend, Dani, remembers her as being in some ways almost autistic. In hindsight, Amanda now wonders whether Syn might have had some form of Asperger's syndrome, which can result in difficulties in social interaction and nonverbal communication. This was, Amanda says, never diagnosed, but she now believes it might have influenced Syn's unique take on life.

She believed she understood things in a way no one else did: was playing a game where no one else understood the rules. She built up a facade of invincibility. Yet behind that there was undoubtedly some degree of self-destructiveness.

So, yes. This was, indeed, failing of sorts on Syn's part. Though if it is failing, it is a common enough one. It is shared by many who have tried to obtain treatment on the NHS, and any reasonable system should make allowances. Instead of looking to catch individuals out and sending them back to square one if they don't give *all* of the right answers, the NHS should be doing more hand-holding, more helping people through a maze entirely of its own creation.

That much, I think I understood even before talking with Syn's friends and family. Less understood was just how significant this would prove, or how helpless, how devastated it would leave Syn feeling.

Against this, it would be wrong to think of Syn as wholly passive. She was, within the confines of her own world – the London club scene, the fast-living queer and trans society – a star: 'an intoxicating goddess that had entire clubs falling over themselves wanting to speak to her'. She had a massive following online, and it seems likely she made real change, real impact on many people's lives.

And that Syn confidence! Or recklessness. It is hard to decide which. One story, though, from when she was staying with Sonny sums up her capabilities. She was on her way to London. Sonny had already taken her to the railway station. But ten minutes later, she was back at Sonny's door. She had forgotten her handbag, her money. So she had persuaded some random guy to give her a lift from the station and – even more incredible – to wait while she picked up her stuff and then take her back again.

Flawed. Amoral? No: she had a moral code of her own. But being as analytical as she was, she had little time for many of the hypocrisies of social convention.

She also, I now suspect, was let down by not being identified as trans much earlier; or rather, by that option not being on the à la carte when she first began to express concerns over her gender. On the one hand, she was lucky – amazingly so – to have gone to a school that had no issues with her defying gender norms, or coming out as gay to all and sundry.

Yet, in the final analysis, she was not so lucky. For most of her teenage years she was unaware of the alternatives or, if she was aware of them, these were filtered through a very particular gay lens. She was taught to regard being trans as essentially 'tragic' and not something that any sensible person would be.

And outside of the spotlight, that confidence melted. She became, as Joey described her, an 'incredibly cute vulnerable kitten'.

So she found a particular scene and a particular set much more closely aligned to the G in LGBT – and within that, much more aligned with chemsex; and so she set out on the road that was eventually to prove fatal. We will never know what 'might have been'. Yet in a world where options are set out clearly and teenagers are helped to find themselves – as opposed to the current quasi-competition in which some ideologues seem more interested in claiming trans people 'for the gay side' – things might have been different.

At the very least, Syn would have encountered other individuals looking to thread a difficult path through the NHS. She might have received better advice much sooner.

The second place where I have changed my mind, perhaps radically, is in the relationship of trans people with society at large. As someone successfully transitioned and that, courtesy of an unexpected inheritance, I managed with few of the issues that Syn faced, and I have to some degree buried my own personal outrage.

Reading behind Syn's story, I feel a rekindling of anger at the fact that for no good reason society treats people like this. Trans people are viewed as a bunch of weirdos whose lives must always be managed and overseen by the wise non-trans majority.

Standards. Pathways. Protocols. Whatever happened to putting the patient first? Why, as Dr Webberley observes, are GPs/GICs so hung up on long assessment periods? Perhaps these make sense with younger, more vulnerable patients. But for adults who have married (and divorced), had children and careers, just what are these meant to prove? Different patients have different needs, from full transition to hormones only: so why is the medical establishment still insisting on a mostly one-size-fits-all approach.

Total trans apartheid is unsustainable. But we need to cease to be the playthings of other powerful interests. 'Experts' still aim to define us, to say that unless we conform to this or that model of behaviour, we are not trans.

Take, for instance, the issue of self-medication. Syn, and many of her friends, self-medded. There is no doubt that this is not an ideal way forward. Drugs obtained on the internet will not necessarily be what they claim to be. Either in strength – or even actual content. In addition, while the risks associated with self-medding are not as high as the risks associated with some forms of drug abuse, they exist.

Individuals taking hormones need to be monitored and supported: that is clear. Yet too often, the response of the wider medical community is punitive and unhelpful. Trans people going in for treatment are warned that they may have their hormones summarily withdrawn; they learn, early on, of the barriers put in place to deny them treatment. They start from a position of unique mistrust in the medical community that is supposed to be helping them.

Yet expertise exists in the community. My own story is part example of that: because I was lucky, able to pay for much of my own treatment and as result to select here and there which pieces of treatment I needed when I needed them.

It is not as though no models exist elsewhere. In Canada, in Australia, trans people are increasingly 'doing it for themselves', with the support of the medical establishment and under an 'informed consent' model light years away from what is on offer in the UK.

Synestra is no longer with us, but her story is not over. For Amanda De Courcy, a lack of understanding across the whole community played as much a part in her death as the drugs. She also feels that barriers to parental involvement, once Synestra was 18, and an independent adult, introduced too much rigidity into the narrative. She believes that more education is needed, and she is working now to bring that about through a charity – Synestra's Community Interest Company – that will aim to provide greater information and support to trans children in schools.

Synestra is not forgotten.

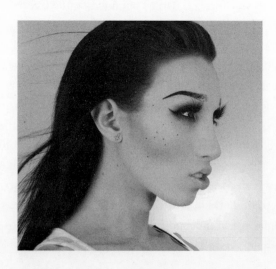

Further Resources

If you are a young person struggling with your gender identity, or your child is suffering with the same, there is an NHS service available for children and young people up to the age of 18. The service will not accept self-referrals. However, your GP, child and adolescent mental health service (CAMHS) team or other healthcare professional can help to secure this for you. The service operates within England only. The Tavistock and Portman GIDS service can be found online at http://gids.nhs.uk

In Wales, the approach is very similar to that in England, and a successful referral, which must be via CAMHS, will eventually end up at the Tavistock.

In Scotland, young people should go to the Sandyford Young People's Gender Clinic in Glasgow (Tel: 0141 211 8618). They can self-refer or be referred by a parent, medical professional, education professional or youth worker.

In Northern Ireland, all GIDS referrals must first go through CAMHS. Details on the services in Northern Ireland are available at http://transgenderni.com/healthcare

In addition, if you would like further information about the issues raised in this book, or are looking for help with your own personal journey, the following may be of help.

Organisations
ClinicT
...is a sexual health service for anyone who identifies as trans, non-binary or gender variant (partners are welcome too). The clinic runs monthly.

Helpline: 01273 523388
Contact form: http://brightonsexualhealth.com/contact-us
Website: http://brightonsexualhealth.com/service/clinic-t

CliniQ

...is a holistic sexual health and well-being service for all trans people, partners and friends. Trans led.

Helpline: 020 3315 6699
Email: n/a
Website: https://cliniq.org.uk

Gendered Intelligence

...works with the trans community and all those who impact on trans lives, and specialises in supporting young trans people aged 8–25.

Telephone: 020 7832 5848
Email: http://genderedintelligence.co.uk/contact/email
Website: http://genderedintelligence.co.uk

GIRES

...is a UK-wide charity with international reach whose purpose is to improve the lives of trans and gender-diverse people of all ages, including those who are non-binary and non-gender. GIRES provides policies, training, e-learning and literature, much of which can be accessed via its website. The charity also maintains a directory of more than 400 trans support groups: www.TranzWiki.net

Telephone: 01372 801 554
Contact form: www.gires.org.uk/contact-us
Website: www.gires.org.uk

LGBT Health and Wellbeing Edinburgh

...was set up in 2003 to promote the health, well-being and equality of lesbian, gay, bisexual and transgender (LGBT) people in Scotland. It provides support, services and information to improve health and well-being, reduce social isolation and stimulate community development and volunteering.

Telephone: 0131 523 1100
Email: admin@lgbthealth.org.uk
Website: www.lgbthealth.org.uk

Mermaids

...provide direct support and information for trans and gender-diverse children, young people and their families, and work to raise awareness amongst professionals and the general public.

Helpline: 0344 334 0550
Email: info@mermaidsuk.org.uk
Website: www.mermaidsuk.org.uk

Pavilions

...provides adult drug and alcohol services for Brighton & Hove. Support is available to anyone concerned about their drug or alcohol use, or for the families and carers supporting those struggling with substance misuse.

Helpline: 01273 731900 or 0800 014 9819
Referrals: referrals@pavilions.org.uk
Website: www.pavilions.org.uk

Terrence Higgins Trust

...is the largest voluntary sector provider of HIV and sexual health services in the UK, running services out of local centres across Great Britain.

Helpline: 080 8802 1221
Email: info@tht.org.uk
Contact form: www.tht.org.uk/our-charity/Footer/Contact-us
Website: www.tht.org.uk

Scottish Transgender Alliance

...works to improve gender identity and gender reassignment equality, rights and inclusion in Scotland.

Telephone: 0131 467 6039
Email: info@scottishtrans.org
Website: www.scottishtrans.org

Further reading

How to Transform Your School into an LGBT+ Friendly Place: A Practical Guide for Nursery, Primary and Secondary Teachers. Elly Barnes and Anna Carlile. Jessica Kingsley Publishers.
LGBT+ inclusion is not part of standard teacher training or induction, which makes it difficult for schools to provide inclusive learning environments and support for LGBT+ pupils. Drawing on an Ofsted and DFE recognised 'Best Practice Award Programme', this book provides everything you need to know about making your school an LGBT+ friendly place.

LGBTQI Parented Families and Schools: Visibility, Representation and Pride. Anna Carlile and Carrie Paechter. Routledge Critical Studies in Gender and Sexuality in Education.
This is a book about the experiences of LGBTQI+ parents and their children, and their relationships with schools. It includes chapters on theories of LGBTQI+ parenting, school inclusion strategies, school policies and the representation of LGBTQI+ parents in the media. Central to the book are the voices of the LGBTQI+ parents and children we interviewed: theirs are stories of resistance, resilience and dignity.

To My Trans Sisters. Charlie Craggs (ed.). Jessica Kingsley Publishers.
An empowering, heartfelt collection of letters from celebrated trans women addressed to those who are transitioning. Each letter offers honest advice from their own experience on everything from make-up and dating, through to deeper subjects like battling dysphoria and dealing with transphobia.

Trans Britain: Our Journey From The Shadows. Christine Burns (ed.). Unbound.
A comprehensive account of the emergence of the trans community in Britain over the last fifty years in particular, featuring eye witness accounts by both trans people and some allies who were present at various milestones. The book is designed to be accessible to non-trans readers, providing a clear timeline and context to understand how and why the community is where it stands today. It is billed as 'everything you always wanted to know about the background of the trans community but never knew how to ask'.